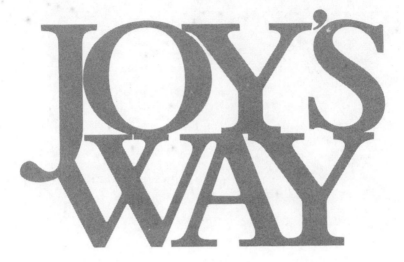

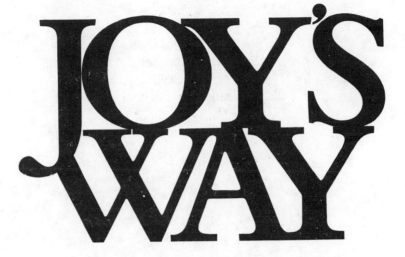

JOY'S WAY

A Map for the Transformational Journey

An Introduction to the Potentials for Healing with Body Energies

W. Brugh Joy, M.D.

J.P. Tarcher, Inc.
Los Angeles

The publisher wishes to thank
Richard S. Gunther
for his active help in making possible
the publication of this book.

Illustrated by Jan Harlow
Design: John Brogna
Manufactured in the United States of America

Published by J. P. Tarcher, Inc.
9110 Sunset Blvd., Los Angeles, Calif. 90069
Published simultaneously in Canada by Macmillan of Canada
70 Bond St., Toronto, Canada M5B 1X3

Q   10   9   8   7   6

To my two outer Spiritual Teachers:

Lona Brugh Joy —
    who bore me, taught me
    Love, gave me nourishment,
    and implanted seeds of heresy.
Eunice Jean Hurt —
    who awakened me with Love
    and ripened the seeds of
    heresy.

CONTENTS

Deep Acknowledgment —
  Tamara Comstock — gifted editing and transcription
  Carolyn Conger — soul support
  Jan Harlow — cover design and illustrations
  Five hundred conference participants at Sky Hi Ranch,
    September 1975–January 1979 — confirmation of the
    Transformational Process
  Wentzle Ruml III — further translation and editing of
    linear and nonlinear material

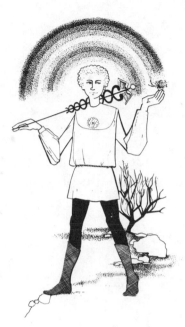

The Fool

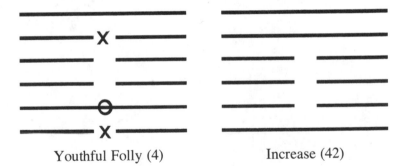

Youthful Folly (4)   Increase (42)

"To strengthen what is right in a fool is a holy task."
I Ching/Book of Changes
Wilhelm/Baynes

Joy is the most
infallible sign of the presence of God.

Teilhard de Chardin

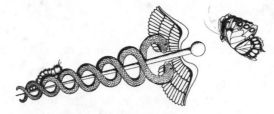

Approaching
the
Transformational Process

On the first of January 1974, at the age of thirty-four, I was a highly successful and respected Los Angeles physician, an internist specializing in lung and heart diseases. By that autumn, in response to an inner voice, I had left the practice of orthodox medicine and, in search of understanding, was traveling the world on an itinerary that included the Findhorn community in Scotland, the Great Pyramid in Egypt and treks in India and Nepal.

Since September 1975, at a ranch in a remote part of the Upper Mojave Desert in California, I have been conducting Conferences on what I call the Transformational Process. More than five hundred people have now had this training, and thousands have heard me speak about it in lectures and symposia all over the country. In the process, the Conference experience has become clear enough in my mind for me to write about it and, I trust, make it still clearer.

I write at this time because I am at a turning point in my life. While Conferences continue to be important to me, I sense that I am about to go through another major transformation, the latest in a long series of them. In a quite literal, though not physical, sense, I am dying; and, in the same literal sense, I am being reborn. I am leaving my present life and going into a new phase.

This book, therefore, marks an end and a new beginning. Being about the Transformational Process, it is a sort of cosmology, it is a partial autobiography insofar as my personal transformations have contributed to the development of the subject, and it is to some extent a do-it-yourself or how-to book.

All my transformations have been of my own choice; I have not lost but gained in changing from the very orthodox, very respectable young physician to the human being now on the verge of giving up his present life, and I wouldn't have it any other way. You are welcome to come along on the journey as far as you wish and are able. The transformations — the ones I have had, the ones you can have — are what this book is all about. The material is fascinating, terrifying to some people and, quite realistically, not without danger. In reading the book — in coming along on the journey — you become a counterpart of the more than five hundred people who have worked with me in Conferences at Sky Hi Ranch.

For a moment now, let's look back at that young physician in 1974.

His academic background and training were of the best. After undergraduate work (completed in 1960) and medical school (1964), both at the University of Southern California, he went to Johns Hopkins Hospital for his first-year internship and first year of residency in internal medicine (1964-66) and to the Mayo Clinic for two more years of residency in internal medicine (1966-68). As an undergraduate he had been elected to Phi Beta Kappa, the undergraduate academic honor society; as a medical student he had been elected to Alpha Omega

Alpha, the medical-school academic honor society; and as a practicing physician he was a Fellow of the American College of Physicians and of the American College of Chest Physicians. He had been commended by the admiral of the Eleventh Naval District for his services at Balboa Naval Hospital in San Diego, California (1968-70), and from 1970 to 1974 was on the staff of the Hospital of the Good Samaritan in Los Angeles and was an assistant clinical professor of medicine at the University of Southern California. He had a large, prosperous and growing practice. All in all, he had what most physicians of his age dream of.

What could ever move such a physician to drop it all and venture into the unorthodox and tainted, perhaps downright scandalous, areas of spiritual and psychic healing? What sent him traveling through Europe, Egypt, India and Nepal for a period of nine months? And what prompted him to return to the California desert to open a center for people to gather to unfold and share his new ideas?

And, you are entitled to wonder, who are the people who have come there to these Conferences on the Transformational Process? A sampling of the first five hundred would include psychologists, psychiatrists, physicians, nurses, lawyers, accountants, chiropractors, psychics, yoga teachers, business executives, movie and television personalities, housewives, jewelers, marriage and family counselors, social workers, artists, writers, dropouts, drug pushers, prostitutes and ministers of every major faith. In this diverse group of people, the Transformational Process brought about deep and fundamental changes in each person's perception of reality and in his or her ability to touch, feel and experience what can only be described as natural, expanded states of consciousness.

In this book I will attempt to express in a collage of words the experiences, both internal and "objective," that have transformed my life. The many ideas and techniques will be presented in a sequence similar to that of a Conference. We will initially develop basic ideas and then move to greater elaboration and application. The concepts and techniques are not in the historical order in which they occurred to me but rather in the functional order that I have found most successful in presenting them. I have included the personal, autobiographical material merely to illuminate the principles, to show how they developed, not where or when or how they fit into the rest of my life.

Because events in my reality, in *real* reality, happen in their own time, their own sequence, their own cause and effect (if any), I am giving this book its head, allowing its structure to unfold as it wishes to unfold. What matters is not the linear, sequential ordering of the incidents that have taken part in my transformation but the new experiential dimensions that come about — where the supposedly solid human body turns out to be an intricate interweaving of energy fields; where disease is not an entity but rather a fixated warp of energy interactions; where the experience of Unconditional Love transcends the limitations of personal love; where mortality itself dies — and becomes immortality — and where I accept the Divine nature of all life forms, simultaneously physical and nonphysical, structured and nonstructured, existing and not existing in any particular form at any given moment.

Only the rational portion of my consciousness demands sequential information; the nonrational portions find such organization tedious, slow motion, superfluous, perhaps even counterproductive to higher levels of comprehension. Therefore, each chapter has essential information to transmit that may or may not be related to the immediately preceding or the immediately succeeding chapter. Even paragraphs within a chapter may not be directly related to their neighbors. They are to be just glimpses, and it is only after many such glimpses that the diversity of my work and the whole extent of the exploration can be grasped — even, perhaps especially, by me. Please bear with me. Enjoy the desultory play of concepts. It is only the outer mind that conceives and perceives sequentially; our essence needs neither time nor sequence. So relax and allow me to unrein the myriad ideas and discoveries I have to share with you.

I will also not give here a detailed description of who or what I am: as the book develops, more of my nature will become apparent. To try to present myself in one or two paragraphs, or even in a chapter or two, would be ludicrous. No human being can be so described, despite our conditioned beliefs to the contrary. Like you, I am a personal collective. Which of the many trained and untrained personifications of our makeup is displayed in any given moment depends entirely upon the circumstances of that moment. Let me share many moments, show many sides of myself, and something in your awareness will synthesize this information into your own unique perspective of me in this book just as you would do in ordinary life. Who or what I am makes no real difference, so long as the insights I give strike some resonating chords in you. It is not your awareness of me that I intend to influence but your perception of reality.

You will find me equally vague, perhaps irritatingly so, in some of my vocabulary. There is, however, good reason for this vagueness. Part of the Transformational Process involves going from the left brain, where words are thought to be understood, to the right brain, where they are not. To talk or write about phenomena that are beyond the left brain, words are, unfortunately, all we have, and they can only approximate these matters from outside their realm. For just one example, I offer the word *Beingness*. It looks a lot like the word "being," and in fact it means everything that "being" means—and more. Where your being is largely restricted to the everyday reality, your Beingness is you on *all* levels of reality. Among the other odd words and phrases you will find here are *impress* and *form nature*. Because they, too, are beyond the left brain, these words are truly undefinable. If as you read this book you pay attention to these words and just let them come to you, you will find eventually that you understand them and know what they mean—and you will still be unable to define them. Because they so closely resemble ordinary words in our regular, left-brained vocabulary, I am going to try to indicate them, the first time each word or phrase appears, with *italics*, and in some cases I will give you some specific hints about meanings.

I expect to mention a number of people in the course of my text. About some of them, but not all, I will add identifying or explanatory remarks. You will probably recognize a few of the names, but some will be unknown to you. Most of them have published, some in readily accessible books and periodicals; others are available only in specialized bookstores, while still others have published their work only in journals. A few have not been published at all. All these people are on the frontier of the new consciousness (and *consciousness* is one of those words that mean more here than they do in the ordinary world of the *outer mind*) and so are worthy of your attention.

And I offer a special note on reports and publications in general. The ones I cite are usually given only as corroboration of my points. They run parallel to what I say, and they certainly do not contradict it; but I do not claim that they prove my statements. The further along I go, the less I think it possible to prove anything.

As an orthodox practitioner of medicine I was confident of the godly attributes of science, secure in my ability to follow behavior patterns currently accepted as normal and dedicated to the belief that billions of men, women and children are innocent victims of diseases that only science and the intellect can combat effectively. Now, as an awestruck, deeply moved individual, I see hard, "objective" reality as an ambiguous realm, filled with the miraculous and unlimited in potential, in which science is only one type of scaffolding, one of many structural frameworks the human mind has conceived in trying to understand the phenomena of life.

Science is only one of the scaffoldings. There are others, equally detailed, that serve as similar aids to understanding — the various frameworks found in religion, metaphysics, psychiatry, psychology, philosophy, law, politics, economics and so on. Each tries to organize reality into coherent patterns of hypotheses called theories, creeds, dogmas, laws and beliefs. In truth, all are merely ideas about life, and all fail to stress their basically hypothetical nature.

The release out of the hypothetical foundations on which all systems of belief rest is the crux of the Transformational Process. We start out entrapped in hypotheses that we believe to be absolute truths. Then, in our transformation, we see that they are only temporary structures capable of teaching only relative truths and, for that matter, that the relative truths are true only in the context of their organizing ideation. The transformation opens vistas of human awareness that cannot be comprehended from any one particular perspective.

Transformation enlarges the context of reality. The awareness is lifted up into states of consciousness where the multidimensional nature of existence is perceived, not just conceived; where it is experienced, not just imagined; where each dogma and each absolute truth is seen as but a single facet of a superconscious whole called Beingness. In the totality of Beingness there is no absolute anything — no rights or wrongs, no higher or lower aspects — only the infinite interaction of forces, subtle and gross, that have meaning only in relationship to one another. Absolutes are concoctions of our rational minds. Reality must never be confused with concoctions. The Transformational Process, the release from fixed beliefs, allows the fragmented awareness to meld into universality.

In this book you will find much discussion of *body energy* and *energy fields*. As you may already suspect, body energy has nothing to do with the food you eat, and energy fields do not involve the kinds of energy that drive motor cars, household appliances and diesel engines. There is some relationship to light, magnetism and electricity; but the relationship is not of any conventional, scientific kind.

Our deepest energies are not located in the head or the body, where most people think they are. From my own rather extensive experience with them — and from corroboration by others, including the more than five hundred participants in my Conferences — I am certain that our energy fields not only interpenetrate the entire physical body, but also extend for some distance around it.

The *chakras* are the centers for these energies, both inside the body and immediately outside it. Known for many thousands of years in Eastern philosophy, the chakras are considered mysteries in the West and, perhaps as a part of their mystery, they still do not appear in many current, standard American dictionaries. They form a nebulous energy complex, composed of major and minor centers, whose activity emanates from specific areas of the physical body. The chakra system is inextricably associated with the form and function of the physical and less physical bodies and with the various states of awareness. Tapping these energies — going into the deep, latent energies from the ordinary, "objective," workaday world — is a radical departure from what is, for most of us, usually normal. Tapping these energies is fire, and the consequences are serious and can be dangerous.

Those individuals who have not worked through ego trips or power trips in relationship to other human beings and those individuals who cannot allow sweeping changes to occur in their lives as a consequence of coming into contact with the information about the Transformational Process should not attempt the techniques described in this book. Every soul is responsible for its own experience. Part of maturation is the ability to draw the "honesty cards" about oneself to the forefront of one's awareness in order to decide upon a course of action and the timing of that action. The consequences of immature judgment, of toying with the chakra system, can be psychosis, aggravation of neuroses, acceleration of disease processes and suicide. But the awakening into certain states of consciousness can bestow gifts of such value that they are beyond price, gifts such as the mastery of any or all of the psi phenomena, healing powers not yet recognized by conventional Western science and deep serenity and knowledge of life.

That the chakra system exists is beyond doubt, as I shall demonstrate in the contents of this book. But no one, not one person, knows what it actually is or all of its aspects, and no one has ever known, despite attempts over thousands of years to master this knowledge. My tentative belief is that the chakra system is an interdimensional transducing system capable of being directed by thought and capable of converting matter into various forms of energy, and vice versa, transcending the constraints of time and space.

As the rainbow is produced by the refraction of light through a prismatic structure of countless water particles so that the frequencies that compose ordinary light are splayed, so, too, the chakra system seems to splay out different aspects of some primary energy configuration through the body. This analogy is heightened by the way that some clairvoyants perceive these force centers and their emanations as constantly changing colored lights, like the light seen streaming through stained-glass windows. My stepping stones into this rainbow are the events that led to my current understanding of the chakra system and to the levels of awareness associated with these forces.

This book isn't intended to please. It is intended to tilt you from the limited possibilities for experience that you now have, no matter how wide open you may think they are, to a set of possibilities that is truly without limits. This book is offered to those who are ready to begin the awakening process, who know at the deepest level of their awareness that they are ready for change from unfulfilling, culturally conditioned life patterns into states of consciousness that commit them to a path of self-realization, who are beginning to become aware that their ultimate limitations are nothing but the restrictions set by their own minds.

I did not want to write this book, nor do I especially enjoy sitting down to compose it. Words are not the same when written as when spoken. An expression of the face or a simple gesture of the hands, combined with careful modulation of the voice, can accomplish in seconds what may take hours to get across in written words. How did I ever happen to select an incarnation where the verbal form of communication is so predominant? Why not a time when telepathic communication transmits instantly what we, as humans in our present time, must belabor and imperfectly reproduce through language? I would much rather be exploring the world or a group of people, meditating or teaching than to be writing a book. Why, then, am I doing it?

I am writing the book because of a recent dream I had and because of an inner voice that won't let me take my usual afternoon nap. The dream, at least the part that I remember, was the signing of my own medical chart. As I was reviewing it to write a summary, I noticed that the chart was not organized — laboratory slips were out of place, and the normal order of the chart was markedly disturbed. I reordered the chart and then signed it. The signature required was peculiar, because my name was given as Joy, William Brugh, M.D., instead of William Brugh Joy, M.D. It reminded me of signing a death certificate. Over to the right of my name was an asterisk and the words *See box above* and the box above commanded: PLEASE HURRY! — in capital letters and red pencil, no less!

The interpretation of this dream was obvious to me. All the material of the Transformational Process has come to me through meditation, through dreams or through inspired states of consciousness when traveling or while working with groups. In group work the information was shared, developed and strengthened, and I gained greater insight into it with each succeeding Conference. But, because I work spontaneously, no two Conferences were the same, nor was the same emphasis placed on the different aspects. Both as it came to me and as I have presented it in the past, the material was disorganized, like the chart in the dream, and it needed to be clarified and written in summary form.

The dream further represents the rounding out — the death — of the initial phase of my work in the Transformational Process. The urgency to complete the book (PLEASE HURRY!) comes from somewhere far within my Beingness, because another, deeper aspect is to be developed in the near future. It is time for me to die in this aspect of my work and to be reborn into another one.

The voice that interrupts my afternoon naps is even more interesting. During Conferences I rise at four in the morning and often work till ten or eleven at night, and I find that a nap from two to four in the afternoon is extremely balancing. Several afternoons ago, as I was about to go to sleep, the entire eleven-chapter outline popped into my head, and at the same time I heard a voice that ordered me, in no uncertain terms, "Get out of bed and write down the overall organization of the book!" I tried to ignore it, but the impulse and *impress* were relentless; and so I got up and wrote down the images I had seen. Then, instantly, I was able to sleep.

Today, as I was about to go to sleep, the book began to take shape. I was in twilight sleep, but simultaneously I was aware that I was dictating the introduction, the material repeating itself over and over again in my own mind. I tried to bargain with my consciousness, telling it that I would begin after I had rested.

My consciousness would not bargain. It is now twenty minutes later. Unable to fall asleep, I have commenced. It flows easily. As I complete one paragraph I see or hear the words for the next one.

I am ready to allow the completion of this phase of my life.

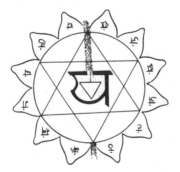

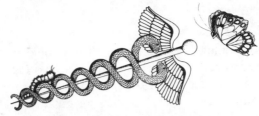

CHAPTER ONE

Basic Concepts

*The subtle exploration into
the obvious is the awakening process.*

Although I am clearly merging into multidimensional aspects of human consciousness, I am only six years into the process, and therefore it is as a beginner that I wish to share what I have experienced thus far. For you to share this strange and wonderful experience with me, it will help for you to work from the viewpoint of a "beginner's mind."

This concept came to the West with Zen Buddhism, but even now few people really comprehend it. With instruction, however, it is invaluable in helping people of all levels of education, social background and religious training to meet any new concept or even to deal with old concepts encrusted in judgments or belief systems. A beginner's mind is that unencumbered, open, allowing, alert, receptive state of consciousness that experiences any and all things with the freshness usually directed only to the totally new. If, for example, an experience is one that a person has had before, all memory that

13

is even remotely associated with it is held in check and not allowed to color the present moment's savoring and exploration of an action, feeling or thought. The moment's interaction is then allowed to sparkle in its originality and multifaceted aspects. In the beginner's mind, *nothing* has ever happened before.

In Conferences, I usually demonstrate the phenomenon of the beginner's mind in two ways—first with the playing of a musical composition. From the ranch library of more than five hundred different selections in every taste and style of music, it is usually fairly easy to find a record that is unknown to most and perhaps all of the Conference participants. Some likely examples are Dvorak's *The Golden Spinning Wheel*, Vivaldi's *Gloria* and Hovhanness's *Mysterious Mountain*. (A fourth selection, which teaches the freshness of the unfamiliar and then strikingly demonstrates what happens when a reactivated memory pattern colors and distorts experience is Rossini's *William Tell* overture. The entire composition is less than twelve minutes long, but most people have heard only the end of it. After the unfamiliar and beautiful music of the beginning, members of Conference groups almost always break into laughter when it suddenly turns into the highly energetic theme of "The Lone Ranger" of radio and television fame. To the beginner's mind, *all* of the overture would simply be musical vibrations of varying intensities and rhythms.)

When I play one of these pieces for the first time, Conference participants find it captivating and exciting and, as I said, usually unfamiliar. If I play it a second time, they may hear most of it, but they are already beginning to anticipate the "good" parts and to exclude the other parts from their listening awareness; at intervals their minds begin to drift. If I then play it immediately for a third time, most of them are bored with it; of what is presented to the ear, they hear about half, or even less. Psychologists call this process "habituation," and it is the very aspect of human consciousness that the beginner's mind attempts to overcome.

Whatever its mechanism may be, habituation's effect is a

filtering of sensory awareness. In such sequences of events, science can demonstrate that the entire sensory input normally reaches the brain. (It does not matter whether the medium is music or even which sense is used.) We must infer, therefore, that the filtering takes place somewhere between the receptive centers of the brain and the awareness of the individual.

Now, taking the final step, we come to a devastating realization: whether of music or anything else, the initial experience is also filtered; only a small portion of *any* total experience reaches our awareness. In effect, our ordinary consciousness is asleep. It is so highly filtered by past conditioning — cultural, personal, or whatever — that, by the time it reaches our awareness, the actual sensory *impress* is highly distorted. The approach through the beginner's mind is an attempt to bypass the filters in order to open the awareness more fully to experience.

When I conduct this habituation experiment with a Conference group, I ask the participants, after each playing of the selection, to express what they have experienced. After the first listening, they report liking or disliking the music and describe the images that appeared to them or the sensations they felt in their bodies. (People's reactions, predictably, are often more about themselves than about the music.) At this point I have not yet talked to them about the beginner's mind; and when I repeat the selection for a second and a third time, most people become a little resentful that I am belaboring the obvious point about just listening to the music. But when I then present the concept of the beginner's mind, explain habituation and the filters of consciousness and play the identical music for the fourth time, most of them report afterward hearing not only sounds of exquisite subtlety, but also passages and instruments they did not remember having heard even on the first listening. The music becomes multidimensional, freshly experienced and more fully appreciated. With respect to this one piece of music on this one occasion, we have bypassed some of the filters.

I then ask the participants to look at and to experience a friend or spouse who may be attending the Conference with them and try to comprehend how much they are really experiencing of that person they think they know so well. Naturally, they are not so proficient in the beginner's mind as to be able to see readily all the aspects of the familiar person, but the point is made. And so the journey into greater awareness can begin. Try it.

Here I am reminded of a statement by Arthur C. Clarke in his *Tales of Ten Worlds*, which John C. Lilly, M.D., quoted in *Simulations of God*: "The person one loves never really exists, but is a projection focused through the lens of the mind onto whatever screen it fits with least distortion." The person you love is only part of the person you see. The person you hate is only part of the person you see. *Anything to which you react is only a part of the anything that is there.* And the person you love, the person you hate and the anything to which you react are all projections from within you. As I tell people in Conferences, even if you were to see an individual as fully as possible with your ordinary awareness, you would still see only a fraction of what could be seen from heightened states of consciousness.

But first things first. The initial task in awakening is to begin to ask whether there is more to experience in any given moment; then to conceive that there may be more; then to experience it; when it is experienced, to conceive that there may be more; and thus go into the cycle again indefinitely. Full mastery of this technique takes years, but, of course, partial mastery is a step in the right direction. It is fundamental to the heightening of awareness at any level of exploration into consciousness.

The second example I use to demonstrate the beginner's mind to Conference groups is myself. I present similar information and experiences to group after group, sometimes with only half a day between the end of one Conference and the beginning of the next, and as I do it I feel the same freshness of energy, excitement and insight as the first time the ideas emerged into my consciousness. After three years of this practice, living with it constantly, I continue to find new aspects in all the concepts. This freshness applies not only to the verbal material but to the music as well.

One question that may occur to you is: he has described some of the attributes of the beginner's mind and has given some examples, but how does one actually achieve the beginner's mind? My reply is: just conceive of it and begin! It is as simple as that. Let it come. It will.

Your outer mind—your everyday "objective" mind—is the very last area of your total awareness to comprehend anything. When it does comprehend in the ordinary sense, it does so only very selectively—along the lines of your racial, cultural, educational, religious and family conditioning. In ordinary reality, we are conditioned beings moving about imitating one another, living in structured ideas about reality, forming a consensual consciousness that constantly tends to verify itself. It may strike your imagination, however, that large groups of people perceive reality very differently, and you may wonder whether anybody has ever experienced what is external to the body without the filtering of awareness.

This wonderment was awakened in me by my nine months of travel in the world after I left my medical practice in 1974. The Europeans, the Egyptians, the East Indians, the Japanese, as large groups, perceive the world through their indoctrination in belief systems peculiar to their cultures as a whole and would defend with great energy their reality systems as the "real" ones. As you explore this phenomenon, you note the division into subcultures, and you begin to see even more subtle subdivisions in villages and towns. What you come to realize is the multidimensional aspect of human consciousness at the level of ideas and conditioning. The cohesive factor in a large group— such as a country or a continent—is a large general belief system or set of ideas about reality, and the same principle goes on to operate in smaller and smaller units. Astonishingly, the ordinary consciousness lives and behaves as if those ideas were reality! Even more astonishing is the ability of the human mind to store many ideas about reality simultaneously and to let them come forth into the outer mind sequentially. Many of these ideas contradict one another, either relatively or absolutely; but the contradictions do not matter in storage, and since they are not emitted simultaneously, the outer mind is blind to the contradictions.

Some brief examples should suffice: most obvious are scientists who, because of their training, demand experimental proof of reality as they have been conditioned to perceive it, but who then may find themselves experiencing — and expressing! — cultural religious attitudes on the Sabbath and never question the fundamental dichotomy between their work days and their religion days; physicians who constantly advise patients on principles of health and disease yet whose personal lives are perfect examples of unbalanced living patterns, who will rationalize and defend both their advice and their lives and will not recognize the contradiction between their two personal belief systems; and religious zealots, whose madness is apt to spring from unconscious attempts to reconcile irreconcilable obsessions, some Divine and some satanic. There are also environmentalists who demand air purification and never give a thought to the styrofoam cups at their meetings; people who are vegetarians on an emotional or spiritual basis but still love leather; and civil libertarians, who favor rights for the radical left and oppose them for the radical right. The shocker here is not that these people embody particular contradictions but the more basic fact that *no* belief systems actually represent reality; they are only structural ideas created out of a small part of the human mind's potential.

If some of the oddball contradictions I have cited are laughable to you, I ask you to consider some entities that you live with every day. Governments, countries, organizations, religions, political parties, businesses, families and many other ''things'' are not things at all but are only consensual ideas that we are conditioned to believe as real. They have no real substantiality and serve only as functions in our societies and our individual lives. When you go to school, to the bank, to work or to a store, you usually go to a specific building, it is true; but the building is not the school, the bank, the work or the store. Rather, it is only a symbolic embodiment of a function: if its function is moved elsewhere, or if the building is used for a different function, the building is given a different symbolic name. From this perspective, the state of California and, for that matter, Sky Hi Ranch do not exist; they are just arbitrary boundaries, enforced by convention, agreement and law. (And the word *ranch*, whether used as a noun or as a verb, is a puzzle all its own. Sky Hi is not a cattle ranch nor even a dude ranch; at Sky Hi we ranch souls.) If you honor your father and your mother, please realize that your father and mother, even if they are still alive, do not exist; the people do, but "father" and "mother" are just names for functions or relationships. And, of course, your own body, however real as a person, is a son or daughter only by sociological consensus.

My point is that, ordinarily, we live not with things but with ideas about things. In many ways this ideation is convenient and valuable, a useful tool in living and communicating with one another; but right now, in the process of our awakening, we must see it as a trap, an automatic, involuntary mechanism that is only a small part of our awareness. Our labels, emotions and prejudices preclude experiencing the full potential of our Beingness. Our ideas about things keep us from perceiving the things themselves.

The *outer mind* is that portion of consciousness that is primarily conditioned ideas about reality. Its awareness is profoundly limited in our attempts to experience what actually exists in any given moment. Like the Pavlovian dog, each individual responds to a cue to which he or she has been trained. A cue can potentially produce many kinds of responses, but to any given cue each individual responds with only one reaction, or at the most a few. In any case, the reaction is potentiated through the mechanism of memory. This limitation of experience is established very early and usually is not altered throughout a lifetime.

The beginner's mind approach asks that the memory be

held in check while an openness to new experience is maintained. The conditioned response is unhooked—separated—from the cue that stimulates it. With this freedom, new growth is possible.

As we begin to fathom this principle, as we begin to use the beginner's mind to see things the way they are rather than the way we have been conditioned to see them, we can also begin to understand the source of the insane consequences of conditioning — wars, destruction, killing, incarcerations, crucifixions, boundaries and so on — of conflicts between belief systems and, even more fundamentally, our all-too-human habit of taking our belief systems as real. From fathoming the same principle, we can also learn to see the magnificence of our creative potential in the rich variations of themes called life, religion, government and so on. The difference between the awful insanity and the creative glory is nothing more than the recognition that belief systems are only belief systems and not realities. *At this level of consciousness we can create anything we desire*, and once we realize that we live only in an idea level of existence that is not based on any intrinsic realness, we may consider the possibility that there are options to our experience and expression of reality. The questioning process brings us naturally, easily and inevitably to the threshold of higher states of consciousness.

Perhaps more than belief systems and conditioning, the emotions, whether consciously perceived or acting subconsciously, seem to be one of the major experiencing mechanisms that dominate the perspective of an individual. Whatever prompts them, emotional responses are undoubtedly valid experiences—that is, they really happen—but we must ask whether the emotional *kind* of response is truly appropriate or whether we have other options of experience either in combination with, or outside of, the emotional-reflex arc.

Does the emotional reflex augment or restrict our appreciation of the life experience? I believe that in the overwhelming majority of individuals emotions are restrictive. The emotional responses are relatively primitive, powerful, reactive experiences that are understood poorly if they are understood at all. I believe that some of the negative qualities of emotion, such as anger, fear, hostility and depression, are functioning properly only when they lead to insight or when they act as a signal to the outer mind that a flaw in perception or in understanding is occurring. This attitude toward the emotions can be appreciated only when we actually know that there are ways to discharge energy other than through emotions, and when we realize that the negative response is a signal from inside and not a fact of reality from outside. Your fear does not mean that there is necessarily a real danger, and your depression does not really mean that you are at the bottom.

The training of a physician illustrates emotional deconditioning and reconditioning and the replacement of the emotional response with other, more appropriate ways to discharge energy. As an undergraduate, before medical school, the student's basic, intrinsic emotional level is conditioned by, and keyed into, the general emotional reaction patterns of his or her family unit, which in turn interacts with the social structure in which the family lives. In medical school the student's pattern of emotional response almost instantly begins to break down, because, with little warning, it is assaulted by the introduction to the dissection of a dead human being, a cadaver. Let me illustrate with details from my own training.

I clearly remember the first day of anatomy class at the beginning of medical school. Each team of four students was issued a body to study for the entire year. The bodies, instead of lying conveniently on dissection tables, were enclosed in plastic bags and stacked on shelves in another room. Each came with the following information: a name, age at death (if known), a brief history of the last illness (which was withheld from us so we could discover during the course of study what events must have taken place to cause the death of our cadaver) and whether the body was willed to the school or was an unclaimed derelict who had died in the skid-row area or in the county hospital. The bodies were saturated with formaldehyde.

To prevent our cadaver's dessication during the year's study, my partners and I had to cart the cadaver over to the dissection room, remove it from the plastic bag, grease the entire body with a substance similar to petroleum jelly and then wrap it with jelly-impregnated gauze, carefully covering each individual finger and toe, the nose and ears, as well as the entire body. Interestingly, all seven women medical students in my class seemed to breeze through this stage without emotional consequences, while five or six of the male students experienced fainting, nausea and vomiting, lightheadedness and other physical reactions to their emotional responses.

Whatever my emotional nature had been before, I knew without question that I was going to have to respond to this experience as much as possible without emotion. My psychological defenses included denial that the cadaver represented a human being like me — it was more like an object of interest and study that reflected a structure similar to my own. And, of course, like all medical students, I defended myself with humor.

My point here is that without control over our emotional nature, we cannot probe or extend our experience of life. The medical student knows that the cadaver is only the beginning of the initiation into the realm of medical science. Still to come are the confrontations with the dying — the dying aged (not too difficult), the dying child (very emotionally charged) and the dying person of twenty to twenty-five (the student's own age, probably the most difficult to encounter) — and then the actual death and postmortem on a person one has cared for medically. During the postmortem examination, the body is not gray, stiff and leathery, as in the anatomy lab. These dead are pale, flaccid and appear to be asleep or drowsing.

My first postmortem was on a child of four. It took every effort of my Beingness not to react to the procedure as my emotions were prompting me to do, but, from a new perspective, I was finally able to study the body and proceed with the postmortem without emotional response. Then I was able to see the magnificence of the death process and the beauty of the lifeless shell of the individual who had animated this form. At that point I became able to understand that my emotional response had been based on my own fears of death and dying, and that those ideas were generated not out of reality but out of stories I had heard or read or seen in movies and out of my reaction to the death of close relatives. The reconditioning of my entire response pattern into a new option when exposed to death or dying was a fundamental experience that gave birth to an important experiential insight: given sufficient motivation, conditioned patterns of response can be altered. The possibility of negative consequences — loss of sensitivity, perhaps suppression, sublimation or even repression — had not yet entered my consciousness, but the positive reward was clear: a beginning mastery over emotional responses could allow me new dimensions of perception that had been previously unavailable or blocked by the emotional expression. This basic insight about the control of the emotions later grew gradually into the concepts of the transmutation of sexual and emotional energies, so that I was able to envision the psychological tools needed to overcome neurosis engendered by repression.

Simultaneously held paradoxical belief systems — contradictions — often pop up in patients or observers in an emergency room. On the one hand, these people admire the physician at work; but on the other, they also condemn the doctor as "insensitive" to what is actually happening, that is, to death, to traumatic injury that may have consequences for a lifetime or to the emotional responses of the patient's family. When people insist that the emotions must be given free expression, I often ask them to relate the consequences of their contention to emergency-room physicians. If these physicians were to react emotionally to the sight of the injured coming in from an automobile accident or a fire, or to the feelings of the patient's family, their use to society would be lost. Physicians who have mastered their emotions (in distinction to those who *repress* emotions) are persons who can, when they choose, express and experience emotion, who have a deeper understanding of what their own emotional nature is and who are capable of sensitive responses to other human beings in times of crisis, rather than cold, icy intellectuals who defend themselves from emotional responses. Note that the key here is that the physician can choose. The more highly developed the individual soul, the greater the number of the options of response.

The first stage of developing mastery over the emotions is holding them in check, either by psychological defense mechanisms or by the technique of identifying with what is called the *witness aspect* of consciousness. (The witness aspect will be covered in more detail later.) Then come the insights and new experiences that feed back into the psyche new response patterns and new understanding, leading eventually to a complete re-evaluation and renovation of the individual emotional pattern. The individual is then capable of acting, rather than reacting.

The following section is intentionally designed to evoke several strong emotional responses conditioned by society. I ask you to keep in the back of your mind the overview that these reactions are centered in culturally engendered ideas about reality and are not the only reactions possible to the given cues. (If aspects of death and dying are particularly distasteful, please proceed to page 28, second paragraph.)

A good example of the variation of emotional responses from a single cue or idea would be different people's reactions to the ideas of cremation or of embalming of the human corpse. First of all, let's emotionally charge the idea even further by using words that elicit stronger reactions. In cremation, we are burning or charring a person who has died, rendering the body to ashes and bony fragments through fire and the use of some blunt instrument. Then, in the West, we usually sweep up the remains into a container to be put into a mausoleum, the ground or the ocean or to be scattered over the earth. In the East, the remains are swept from the burning area directly into water, usually a river.

I would venture to say that most people in the West react negatively and strongly to this kind of treatment of a formerly living human being. I have heard, for example, that it is a sin to cremate a body; that it is primitive and unthinking; that it is ugly and uncaring; that the body must be preserved because at some future time that same body is to return to the same functions as when it was alive; that satanic forces operate when the body is put into the fire; that the process of cremation is inhumane for the departed soul who might have to experience the fire; that it is a desecration of the life form to destroy the body in such a way; that there is no rest for the departed soul when its body is destroyed; and so on. In our Western culture, Jews and Catholics are two large groups that traditionally do not cremate their dead (though their reasons may not be the ones I have cited), and there are millions upon millions of other people to whom the idea of cremation is simply unthinkable.

But to other millions, perhaps even more millions, it is unthinkable to do anything but cremate the body. These people, predominantly in the East, believe that it is necessary to burn the body in order to liberate the soul; that the soul can't leave the body completely until its form is dissolved; that the fire represents the sun or god action or transmutation; that the body is of no real consequence in a soul's journey and development except as a vehicle to be used temporarily and discarded like old clothing at death.

These ideas are certainly startlingly different, but now I want to suggest something that may be equally shocking in a different way. Is it possible that both these polarities — along with the entire intermediate area of response between them — are *equally valid*? Can it be that they depend upon the perspective of the individual rather than upon reality? Is it possible that in truth it doesn't really make any difference and that all these emotional reactions about life and death are based more upon fear and immature thinking than on understanding?

If you are a conventional Westerner, made uncomfortable by the idea of cremation, you may be intrigued by what observers would see if they could follow a body — perhaps yours — from death in the hospital to burial in the cemetery. The usual practice is to attempt to protect bereaved survivors from the reality of death, to make it all seem sweet and gentle.

As soon as a person dies in a hospital, any tubes that were placed into the body — veins, trachea, stomach, bladder or whatever — are removed. The eyes are closed by bringing the lids down with finger pressure; the sheets are usually changed if they are badly soiled; and the blanket and sheet are drawn up to the chin. The arms are placed at the sides or on the chest, and the legs are straightened out. A pillow is placed under the head. Only then is the family allowed to view the body. Later — after the viewing, with the family safely out of the way — the rectum is packed, the penis may be tied with a string to prevent bladder leakage or the vagina may be packed for the same reason. The feet are tied together, the hands are tied together and an identification tag is placed on the great toe. The body is placed on a stretcher and covered with pillows and a large cloth so that it isn't obvious what is being transported through the corridors to the hospital morgue — usually located in the obscurity of the basement or the ground floor. No one, except authorized personnel, physicians or morticians and their aides, is allowed into that section of the hospital. Innocent bystanders must be protected from accidental contact with the realities of death.

The body is stored in a large refrigerator until autopsy or until the mortician is called. Usually, but not always, a white sheet covers the entire body. Rigor mortis, the stiffening of the body, occurs in a matter of hours. It later "breaks" spontaneously, so that by the time the usual autopsy is performed, the body is again flaccid. (If the body is embalmed before autopsy, however, it will have been stiffened by the chemical action.)

If an autopsy is to be performed, the body is removed from the refrigerator and placed on the dissection table, a large, rectangular structure with stainless-steel top and gutters or sloping indentations to catch the body fluids during the dissection and convey them to a sink at the foot of the table. If a full autopsy has been granted by the family, the chest cavity is opened first by an incision through the skin with a scalpel and then with a power saw and chisel to cut away the breast bone, the sternum, to expose the heart and lungs. The incision into the abdomen is carried from the lower part of the front of the chest to the pubic bone.

If the brain is to be examined, then while the pathologist works on removing the organs, an assistant uses the power saw to take off the entire top of the skull in order to remove the brain. Before the skull bone is cut, however, an incision is made from the back of the scalp at the base of the head and is carried up behind each ear so that the scalp can be pulled over the top of the head, thus offering access to the skull. The scalp flap rests over the face. If the brain is not to be examined, the face is usually covered with a cloth.

Every organ is carefully inspected and weighed, and tissue samples are taken, to be mounted on slides for study under the microscope. The eyes and face are usually not touched, nor are the genitalia, legs, feet, arms and hands. After the organs are removed, the spine is inspected from the front, and usually a piece of bone marrow is taken, also from the front, from the lumbo-sacral area.

To help the mortician in the embalming process, the pathologist may tie off all the major vessels that were cut during the dissection — but few pathologists are so considerate. The removed organs are then randomly replaced in the body cavities. (The brain is not put back, but is usually placed in a fluid to "fix" it for several days before it is examined. Before embalming or fixation, the brain is a jelly-like substance, and the fixation process firms it up so that it is easier to handle.) The skullcap is put in place and the flap of scalp pulled back over the head and sutured, closing the body.

When the mortician picks up the body, he places it in a black or dark blue cover sheet or bag and transports it in a windowless black or white truck to the embalming parlor. What happens to it there has been well covered in such books as *The High Cost of Dying* and *The Loved One*. The essence of the mortician's talents is to erase as completely as possible all clues that the person has died. The body is dressed in his or her best clothes. Usually there are no shoes, and only the parts of the

body that are carefully prepared are the ones that can be seen —
the face, the upper torso and the arms and hands.

Next comes the funeral. It is all done with great dignity.
The music is beautiful, the flowers are beautiful, the body is
beautiful and the mourners, however grief-stricken, are left
with the impression, certainly not denied by the mortician, that
the body will remain beautiful forever. Such, unfortunately, is
not the case. Depending on the attention paid by the mortician
and the money paid by the family, the body goes into an
intermediate stage of decomposition in six weeks to two years.
In ten years, the body cannot be considered intact: only the
clothing, the skeleton, the hair, the teeth, fingernails and
toenails and portions of skin remain.

Observing the entire death and disposal process, one gets
the feeling that the person is not really allowed to be dead, held
back not for his or her sake but for the sake of the living left
behind. Even in those of us who know all these facts about death
and dying, our belief systems and the emotional responses they
evoke lead to a rationale that is almost impossible to understand.
Why not present the objective natural aspects of death to our
awareness? Why not let ourselves come into some understanding of the gigantic deception in which we all participate at one
time or another? How can we appreciate reality if we constantly
adulterate it in order to conceal some aspect that is emotionally
upsetting?

Mollifying the emotions, and as a consequence preventing
the experiencing of reality, is a major pattern for much modern
civilization, especially in the West. This unreal reality constantly strives to conceal anything that doesn't fit into the
culture's belief system. People in the East feel that the Westerner is unbelievably body-oriented, to the point of irrationality:
the Western identification of the self with the body — along
with the shrouding over of the actual death process — really
limits our appreciation of the totality of life. I must agree and
state that the culprit in this plot against our perceiving reality is
the unbridled emotional reactions.

Few people realize, or are willing to realize, that the physical body does not die in one brief moment. In the fields of medicine and law there is a major controversy going on over what constitutes death of the body. Science has progressed to the point of sustaining the body without one or more of the major organs — brain, heart, kidneys, adrenal glands, pancreas, most of the gastrointestinal tract, the reproductive organs, spleen, spinal column, the lungs — for varying periods of time, from hours to years, either by using mechanical devices or through organ transplants. Almost all authorities, whether legal or medical, would agree that when the central nervous system (i.e., the brain) is destroyed, legal death has occurred. But actually the body dies over a much longer period of time. Although the brain dies in minutes, the cells that produce hair and nails continue to survive for many months after the person has been buried. Ironically, this cellular death is actually delayed by the embalming procedure, which stops the natural decomposition of the flesh.

At some point in the not too distant future, science will learn how to unlock the mechanism by which a protean, undifferentiated cell turns into whatever specialized cell or cells it is to become. Then it will be possible to take the long-surviving cells from hair or nails and stimulate them into producing entire physical beings. If this differentiation process seems farfetched, please remember that we all begin that way: our physical form appears from a single cell, undifferentiated at conception, with cellular material from the mother's ovum and genetic material from both parents. The work of Dr. Harold Saxon Burr, Ph.D., at Yale University suggests that this developing cell, the zygote, is surrounded by a field of energy that, *independent of the nucleus of the cell*, initiates and controls at least the basic growth axis of the cell. In other words, growth at this stage, despite the hypothesis prevalent in science today, may not be entirely under the control of the genes. Some radical thinkers, including me, even suggest that this energy field constitutes a still more fundamental unit of our Beingness that is subphysical, more fundamental than the physical, perhaps an energy manifestation in the zone between the physical and the nonphysical, an interdimensional link that modern science has not even dreamed about.

Thus we reach the field of physics by way of the protean cell and its energy field. As you may know from even slight knowledge of modern physics, matter is not what our physical senses report it as being. Our senses tell us that our bodies are solid, "real" objects encased in a solid, "real" skin covering. These "realities" are what we experience as our physical selves. We are unaware of our bodies' activities at the cellular level, let alone the molecular and atomic levels, and to approach the subatomic levels and relate them to our own form and structure is mostly intellectual ideation and not in any way experiential. After mystical experiences or hallucinogenic-drug experiences, however, a few people report having felt cellular, atomic and subatomic activities in their bodies. These reports are relatively rare, but what is most interesting about them is that science does not recognize these experiences as valid. In this instance, two specializations subsumed under the general name of "science" hold conflicting belief systems: the biological sciences tell us that we cannot experience what the physical sciences tell us is reality.

Such contradictions and denials are characteristic in science. Prevalent theory at any time is apt to deny even the possibility of something that is just over the horizon. From the ancient Greeks to the present, awareness of the human body has progressed from the level of the gross form and structure to the level of the organ systems, to the cellular level, to the molecular level, to the submolecular level and finally to the atomic and subatomic levels. On these latter levels we don't find matter — we find only swirling or oscillating fields of energy, and between these observable energy interactions we find an unbelievable amount of what appears to be nothingness. The truth is that our bodies — like all "matter" — are composed of a great deal of nothingness and a smidgen of matter or energy interaction. An atomic nucleus and its electrons are both energies, and the distance between them, relative to their sizes, is in proportion to the distance between the sun and the earth. There is a vast amount of nothingness.

In modern physics, one current theory holds that all matter — and, thus, all energy — is actually trapped light. I find this suggestion intriguing, because many mystical and cosmic experiences report light of various colors emanating from all objects. This light appears to be intrinsic to an object, rather than being reflected from the object; that is, the object itself emits the light and can be seen in total darkness. Without even considering the nature of intrinsic light, with all our sophistication, we do not know what ordinary light is. Our understanding of it is still theoretical.

Light and sound are accepted in conventional medicine as energy forces capable of healing. Light, in the many frequencies that we know as colors, has been shown to be effective in influencing certain abnormalities of the body. For example, blue light is used to treat jaundiced infants, and the mechanism is clearly known: the frequency of blue light is capable of breaking up the chemical bonding of the bilirubin molecule and thus converting it into a substance less toxic to the central nervous system. For another example, ultraviolet light is used to treat certain skin disorders and, in sterilization techniques, to kill bacteria and influence virus replication. Sun tanning and sunburn are both produced by light beyond visible frequencies, and when light is produced in a single frequency — as a laser beam — it can make incisions into the body and, outside medicine, can cut metal, fabrics and other materials.

Sound is used in orthodox medicine in the form of ultrasonics — sound frequencies far above the range audible to humans. These frequencies are used to vaporize liquids in inhalation therapy for respiratory patients, in diagnostic equipment which bounces sound waves through the body to produce so-called echograms, and in direct application to the body to promote the healing of injured tissue. Down in the ordinary listening ranges, sound in the form of music is used to soothe or calm supermarket shoppers, operating-room personnel, and office and factory workers. Sonar uses sound waves in the sea in a way analogous to the diagnostic equipment that makes echograms. And I will share some further insights about sound later in the section about high-intensity sound — in the form of music played at high volume — as a tool in precipitating expanded experiences in awareness.

Although we may recognize that sound and light can influence us psychologically, most of us have not conceived that our psychological aspect, like our physical structure, may be nothing more nor less than a configuration of energies. I believe that it is. As I see it, the ''density'' of this psychological energy is far less than the density of what we know as matter, and therefore it is capable of interpenetrating the energy fields that make up matter.

Does this information begin to pique your curiosity as to what we really are? Doesn't it begin to shift your attitude about what is real and what is only apparent? If you can see that a body is an energy interaction, can you also see that a disease must be an energy interaction, too? Isn't it conceivable, then, that there are unexplored combinations of energy interaction that may alter a disease-energy interaction? Could energy fields produced by human thought be among these therapeutic configurations? Could essential thought — thought before it is shaped into language or ideas, images or visions — be more fundamental than matter itself? Could essential thought even originate matter — create it and its counterpart, energy — or at least organize it into forms and structures? What cures is not penicillin or other medicine in tablet or liquid form; what cures is actually a combination of energy forces that is capable of influencing other energy forces. There are many such energy configurations, as yet unknown — or denied by — science that can influence the fields of energy that are manifested as the apparent physical form.

In starting you toward a beginner's mind, I have introduced here only a few basic concepts — enough, I hope, for the average reader to feel tilted out of his or her comfortable belief structure about reality and to begin to enter into dimensions of awareness that are based on scientific probing and personal observation as well as the mystical, spiritual and holistic experiences of reality. I feel that if more information from many belief systems is presented to a developing human consciousness there will be less fantasizing and greater application of our potential as conscious beings.

The whole subject of belief systems always reminds me of the old story about the blind sages examining the elephant. If we allow ourselves to examine only the tail or the trunk or the legs, we come to believe that it is a round tube of varying diameters and we completely miss the unifying pattern. Even worse, we have created an animal that does not exist.

We are all, of course, blinded to some extent by our limitations, and it may be that we will never get rid of them entirely. Insofar as it is possible, however, let us experience the whole elephant.

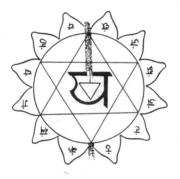

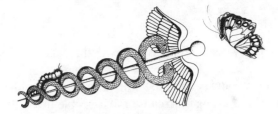

CHAPTER TWO

Teachers, Psi Phenomena
and the
Hologram Analogy

*Some teachers are hallways and some
teachers are staircases; to have breadth and depth in
your expanding awareness, find both kinds.*

In my current work, I repeatedly emphasize that there is but one
basic teacher: Life itself. Life is the great teacher. As we enter
adulthood in the normal pattern, we encounter many varieties of
specialized teachers—e.g., mother and father; brothers; sis-
ters; playmates; the professional teachers we encounter in established educational systems, both public and private; and our
marital partners—but I want to extend the concept of the
teacher to include every human experience. What a specific
human teacher teaches may or may not be true, but all of life's
experiences are intrinsically valid. It is only in our interpretation
of them that there can be potential error.

Generally in our cultural heritage, and more formally in
our educational systems, we are trained or conditioned to conceive of teachers as always being outside us. Any new information, to be valid, either must come from an individual or a
consensus representing authority in a particular area or must be

logically deduced from controlled research based on the scientific method. Any information from any other source is open to question and subject to some degree of invalidation. This sanction is so strong as to cause most people in the West to declare as improbable or even impossible certain experiences that, to a growing but still small number of people in the West, are real and normal. Although most other Western people would deny them, they happen; they do not represent authorities, intellectual or otherwise; they are not derived from experiments or the scientific method; and they are not external. They are internal teachers from experience, from life itself.

I speak of the West in this connection because in many other cultures in the world today people experience life and reality in a different manner—and it is all entirely normal to them. For those people it would be difficult to understand how Western science can deny such basic life experiences as *telepathy* (transmitting and/or receiving through impresses from other conscious life forms), *precognition* (perceiving the future), *past cognition* (seeing, in the present, events that occurred in the past), *psychokinesis* (moving or influencing objects through the power of thought alone), *clairvoyant perception* (seeing events at a distance; often including visions of the auric fields and chakras of human beings and animals), *clairaudience* (hearing sounds or voices at a distance, in the past or the future), *clairsentience* (feeling other beings' emotional responses and/or pains and/or other bodily sensations) and *materialization* and *dematerialization* (making objects seem to appear or disappear either in one's presence or at a distance).

While Western science rejects these phenomena, called *psi phenomena*, my personal experience with them has been too extensive and too deep for me to do anything but accept them. In addition, many individuals with excellent credentials discuss aspects of mind-over-matter phenomena in published reports and public lectures—such men and women as Paul Brenner, David Bresler, Barbara Brown, Elmer and Alyce Green, Valerie Hunt, Shafica Karagulla, Stanley Krippner, Lawrence LeShan, John C. Lilly, Evarts Loomis, Jaquelyn McCandless,

Edgar Mitchell, Richard Moss, Thelma Moss, Kenneth Pel-
letier, J.B. Rhine, Elisabeth Kübler-Ross, James Rota, O. Carl
Simonton, Harold Stone, Robert Swearingen, Charles T. Tart,
William A. Tiller and Jack Zimmerman. Many other people of
academic, scientific and medical standing discuss these subjects
seriously and sympathetically, but the particular people I mention have come to my attention during the past three years. Most
I know personally, and they are all, in my opinion, sincere,
honest and inspired by their investigations and experiences.
Any human being who by now doesn't recognize mind-over-
matter phenomena as valid parts of reality is living in the dark
ages of unenlightened science.

I feel no need to prove the existence of psi phenomena,
either to myself or to other people. A facet of my interest instead
is to develop psi abilities further both in myself and in others,
not as ends in themselves, but as steppingstones into com-
prehensive awareness. How they work and why they work is
less important than the direct experience itself. Actually, questions of how and why often impair the natural tendency to such
experiences. I do know that until one experiences it directly,
either through another gifted human being or through personal
experience, that which is termed psi is only a topic of
conversation—frivolous, intellectual or skeptical—to most
people in Western society. However secure the belief systems
of the frivolous, the intellectual and the skeptical may be, those
people are self-condemned to a limited experience of life.

I believe that human beings in general are currently undergoing a revolution of the most astonishing proportions in the
area of human awareness. This expanded awareness will so
fundamentally alter our perception of time and space, so drastically challenge most current scientific hypotheses concerning
matter and its structure, that it must validate what all religions of
the world claim, the existence of human consciousness in forms
in addition to the human physical body.

I base these statements on my personal experiences. To
me, confirmation or denial from other people or from their
writings is less important than my own direct experience in

these matters. To avoid misrepresenting my own abilities, let me state that I consider my experiences to be only in their initial stages of development. They are often sporadic, and they are usually available to me only when I am working with others, either during workshops or Conferences or in some sort of psychotherapeutic interaction. I am quite sensitive to the emotional patterns present in other human beings, and I am at times aware of their future and past general patterns, too. While I can usually catch the overall trend, it is only rarely, at this stage of my development, that I can see or know specific details about my future or someone else's past or future — or even someone else's current activities. I usually need to talk to a person only briefly before I begin to become aware of things that have not been revealed in our conversation. I have had experiences of clairaudience and clairsentience, both remotely and locally, along with experiences in telepathic rapport.

The majority of my psi experiences have been in the field of the telekinesis of living tissue — that is, in "healing." Remember, however, that I consider *all* psi phenomena as by-products of the development of expanded states of consciousness, whether that development occurs through volition or by "accident." Healing is just one of several psi phenomena, and one must not be seduced into overemphasizing the importance of the ability to heal.

When I direct energy through my hands, pain anywhere in the body is most easily and consistently relieved, whether the pain is of psychological or physiological origin, whether the body is mine or another's. Occasionally, masses have simply disappeared under my hands, and people often report that they feel as if my hands were physically inside them. In the field of clairvoyance rather than telekinesis, I am often aware of what is wrong with another person before my logical mind could possibly deduce the information from facts.

It is most important at this point to say that many times I have been wrong and that other times nothing has happened when I have shared energy through my hands. Baffling as these incidents are, the positive experiences overwhelmingly influence me to continue into deeper explorations.

As subjects for discussion, teachers and parapsychological phenomena belong together. Psi abilities are usually, if not invariably, learned from teachers of advanced, expanded or natural states of consciousness, and a good part of the teachers' own learning comes from parapsychological phenomena. Unfortunately, not all teachers are all that they claim to be — or, often, all that they think they are. Many teachers simply parrot other teachers' work. Good teachers are rare. Excellent teachers of heightened consciousness are jewels. With care it is possible to tell them apart.

I distinguish excellent teachers by several criteria. They are, above all else, *inspired*. Their ideas and their Beingness exalt and uplift anyone who may come in contact with them. They are invariably gifted in one or more of the parapsychological areas. Usually, but not always, they are aware of their destiny from an early age. Their ego structure is clear of major "knots" that would influence their teaching. They are eclectic in their approach to life; they see the underlying patterns in such areas as religion, social structure, life forms and interpersonal relationships. They are visionaries who deeply sense an unfolding evolutionary trend in the human experience. They understand and have resolved the apparent paradoxes and contradictions between the individual and the group. They are able to transmit a perspective that shocks the conditioned mind into surrender to greater awareness. They are able to break their teaching into progressive steps, and they fully realize that statements made to one group of people may be diametrically opposed to statements appropriate to more advanced students. They have resolved the question of light and dark forces, of positive and negative action. They see everything, but they do not judge any action or individual. Committed to a life of service to humankind, or to an even higher order of intelligence, they have little or no need to live in personal relationships. They radiate a quality of Love and understanding that words cannot express adequately. They are knowledgeable in both exoteric subjects and esoteric subjects. They have access, in varying degrees, to *direct knowledge*: they can tap information from levels of awareness other than the usual outer mind or memory, and they can bring this information through without distortion. This process is called channeling, and the teacher is the channel.

There are three major channeling methods. In one, the teacher enters a trance state and appears to have an entity speaking through him or her. The key to this form of channeling is that the teacher is totally unaware of the process and later has no recollection of even the slightest detail of what was said or what action took place during the trance. The channel's voice may be considerably different from normal, as may the cadence and other characteristics of the speech pattern. The channel may take on the movements and characteristics of the opposite sex or may remain relatively motionless, his or her voice monotonous and without inflection. The criterion of this kind of channeling is that the information that is transmitted is usually foreign to the channel's outer ordinary mind.

A good example of a person who used this kind of channeling is Edgar Cayce, who in trances often spoke on subjects that were quite outside the fields of interest and knowledge of his outer mind. In trances, he often saw people at distances, and accurately described what they were wearing and the surroundings in which they were living. His diagnostic acumen was utilized by many orthodox medical practitioners. Time, either past or future, was no barrier to his trance consciousness. His abilities while in trances were mind-boggling; yet when he was not in trance, he suffered all the constraints of ordinary awareness. This point is important to note, because it clearly shows that there are states or levels of consciousness unavailable to even the most gifted teacher when he or she is operating in the logical, conditioned, outer-mind portion of awareness. Pay attention to this aspect, because you cannot always identify even a great teacher when that person is in ordinary awareness. Make your decisions about a teacher when he or she is in heightened consciousness. Otherwise you may entirely misjudge the individual and miss an experience beyond your ability to conceive.

I have met a number of heightened teachers and have read the writings of many others, and they all display a great difference between their heightened awareness and their ordinary common states of consciousness. I am speaking about such persons as Sri Sathya Sai Baba, Bhagwan Shree Rajneesh, Ram Dass, Tarthang Tulku, Baba Muktananda, Eunice Hurt, David Spangler, Franklin Merrell-Wolff, John Lilly and Alan Watts to name a few. Failure to understand this difference has been the source of much criticism directed at each of these teachers by ignorant people who expect them to fit into their own particular belief systems as to how a teacher, saint or avatar must behave twenty-four hours a day. Not one great teacher, now or in the past, has escaped the personality-development phase of human awareness, and most of them have had to spend a large part of their lives in clearing out the clutter of their outer-mind conditioning. Furthermore, no embodied teacher remains in expanded states for indefinite periods of time. Appreciate them when they are, and appreciate them when they are not.

A second form of channeling is the heightened state where the channel "steps aside" and allows another apparent entity to "come through"; in this form, the channel witnesses and hears the entire contents of the material, vocalized or written. Such channels have the sensation that something external to themselves is operating through them. They may not know the significance of the information brought through, but they are awake and aware, like a listener or an observer. I know personally three people who work primarily in this manner, and I have heard of others. One famous person whom I did not know, but who was a prolific writer and an excellent example of this form of channeling, was the late Alice Bailey.

The third form of channeling is more rare and, in my opinion, a more desirable method of channeling. In this form, the channels are fully awake — in fact, superawake. Ideas flow into their consciousness. There is no sensation of something other than self talking through them. They are totally aware of what they are saying while they are speaking, though they may not remember the details after they finish. This kind of channeling requires highly integrated consciousness, because in it the channels' conscious awareness must be heightened to the same level as that from which the information they are expressing and experiencing comes. It may be personal prejudice on my part, but I find that the people who channel in this way are less compartmentalized in their daily lives than those of the two other channeling categories.

Since many teachers use a combination of methods, the divisions in channeling are somewhat artificial and are useful only to learn to note differences in the methods that different teachers use. The all-important point is that, regardless of the method of channeling, the information a teacher brings forth from these higher dimensions of consciousness comes from direct inspiration rather than notes, books or any outside source. Teachers may use established models on which to reflect what they are saying — the Bible, the Cabala, the Vedas — but the essence of the material coming through is inspired, intuitive and strikes deeply those who are exposed to their voices and their writings. There is a notable similarity in the basic teachings of all great teachers, and I think it reflects the fact that they all enter a comparable state of consciousness and that their individuality determines only the discrepancies between them. As astute students know, true spiritual teachers speak a common nonlanguage. Their presence, their voice vibrations, combine to produce this effect. Their words are the least of it.

If you are seeking a higher teacher, let go of any concept you may hold about what such people look like or act like or where they may be found. Many mediocre teachers take on the garb and mannerisms of the spiritual teacher stereotype. Their underlying dynamic is clear: because they are usually insecure, they need external adornment to establish themselves; and thus they gratify undiscerning students who, in their strong desire to find the ideal teacher, end up with only their idea of the ideal rather than with a teacher who is truly great. The truly great have no need to play out a role to meet the needs of their disciples.

Although I have stressed parapsychological abilities as attributes of teachers of consciousness, it is by no means to be construed that a teacher who can foretell the future or past, or who can materialize or dematerialize, or who can heal incurable diseases, is necessarily a great teacher. In fact, psi abilities can be traps for the naive mind, which immediately gives vast power to such a person or makes assumptions far beyond what can be reasonably assumed about the individual who is gifted in these particular areas. It reminds me of the natives in "uncivilized" lands who, on first encountering civilized people, see their guns, flashlights, tape recorders and so on and think that they are supernatural beings.

It is well-known in metaphysical circles that parapsychological gifts, no matter how impressive to untrained persons, are not the criteria of enlightened masters. Enlightened masters, if they use their gifts at all, are fully aware that these feats occur in the phenomenal reality structure and have no great significance in the area of awareness that transcends the physical material world. What matters is not the feats demonstrated but the awareness of the teacher. In fact, if these abilities are all or most of what distinguishes the teacher from ordinary human beings, I suspect that the teacher is trapped in areas of power and control over people — so-called power trips and ego trips. Unfortunately, many people with superficial knowledge of metaphysical teachings can convincingly deny playing power or manipulation games while they continue to misuse these phenomena. Therefore, seekers beware! It is your responsibility to discern your own teacher.

There is a wonderful old saying that comes to mind: "When the student is ready, the teacher appears." The student who is at the initial levels of training will meet the perfect teacher for him or for her at that level.

But here another warning is timely. While the teacher may appear fathomless from the beginner's ordinary consciousness, no teacher ever can be. The mistaken belief may lead not to an expanded development of the soul but rather to a narrowing. When the time comes for further development, the seeker must be willing to release from his or her current teacher, however valuable that teacher has been till then.

An analogy out of my own experience, but not from the field of expanding consciousness, is the rich and varied training

I received in orthodox medicine. I studied not at just one school but at three well-recognized institutions. My medical-school training at the University of Southern California was exceptional in clinical medicine, the part that teaches how to care for the patient; at Johns Hopkins Hospital in Baltimore, Maryland, I learned academic precision, an additional facet that was highly polished; and at the Mayo Clinic in Rochester, Minnesota, I learned balance. Since the three institutions, in regard to a specific medical problem, often had three different, fairly rigid approaches, with diametrically opposed therapeutic concepts, it was an awakening for me to discover that all three achieved positive results. The same holds true for spiritual teachers. Round out your explorations into the barely charted realms of consciousness by experiencing many teachers, not just one.

One last comment on teachers: Eunice Hurt, my own teacher, often said, "Before you give yourself to a teacher, watch to see which way the power is going." When the power is held by the teacher; when the teacher acts like a god or saint or special person and gives little or no instruction to bring the students into the areas from which the teacher is operating; when the teacher begins to seek personal accumulation of material aspects, either directly or by implication; when (though empowering *can* take place through the sexual act) the teacher begins to suggest that the final empowering can occur *only* by going to bed with him or her — then the power is going to the teacher.

When the teacher gives back all power you have delegated to him or her; when the teacher inspires you to your greatest potential, whether it is in your awareness or not; when a teacher loves you, all fellow human beings and all life forms without distinction — then the power is flowing to you.

So far I have been talking about outer human teachers. There are also Inner Teachers — phenomena that I sincerely hope all people will eventually encounter — as well as teachers in the animal, plant and mineral kingdoms. These I will discuss in another chapter, along with my experience with Eunice Hurt, my second teacher, whom I call my awakener or Love made manifest.

To complete this second chapter, certain concepts from the holographic model may be helpful. The hologram is a three-dimensional image that appears in space through the action of light waves interacting with one another. The basic ideas are simple. To record an image holographically, a laser beam of "coherent" light (light of a single wavelength) is passed through a half-mirrored prism, which splits it into two identical beams at right angles to each other. (See figure 1.1) Beam 1 (the "reference" beam) then passes through a lens, which widens it, and goes on to strike the holographic plate or film without ever striking the object being holographed. Beam 2 (the "object" beam) also goes through a lens and is widened. But then it also goes on to strike the object, and part of the light that strikes the object is reflected from the object to the holographic plate. As the reference beam and the object beam meet near the surface of the holographic plate, they interact to form a complex wave pattern, which is imprinted on the holographic film. Unlike ordinary photography, the patterns produced in the film are not of the object holographed but are interference patterns of the two beams striking the surface together. Instead of a picture, the pattern appears in the form of geometric designs; but, with the proper equipment, a laser beam projected through the completed holographic plate will form a three-dimensional image of the object in space rather than a picture on a screen.

In ordinary photography, a screen or some other object must stop the projected image and reflect it back to the viewer's eye; but in holography, no screen is necessary. Light waves interacting with each other produce the image that the eye sees in space.

Theoretical psychology is currently considering the possibility that the appearance of objects in space may be a function of the two sides of the brain, itself forming something like a holographic film, which cognition then organizes into images. With all of our deepening understanding of the modality of vision, we do not understand how light, entering the eye and being transmitted back to the visual cortex is manipulated to make objects appear *outside* our heads. The holographic theory comes closest to a possible solution.

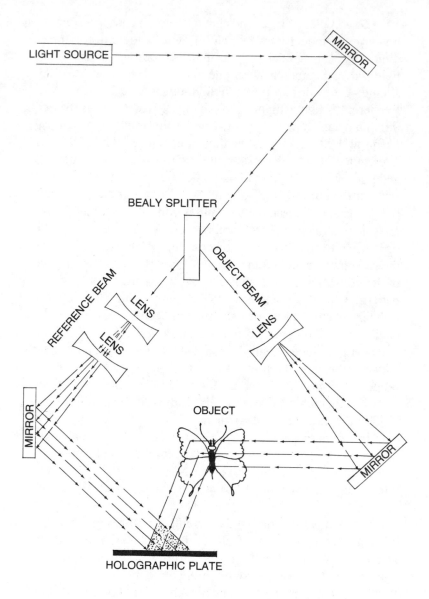

LIGHT SOURCE

MIRROR

BEALY SPLITTER

REFERENCE BEAM

OBJECT BEAM

LENS

LENS

LENS

MIRROR

OBJECT

MIRROR

HOLOGRAPHIC PLATE

Fig. 1.1
Hologram

Far more interesting to me, however, and germane to paranormal or "natural" states of consciousness, is to consider the reaction of the holographic plate or film that records the image of light interference. In ordinary photography, if the negative is cut in half, one piece has half the recorded image and the other piece has the other half. If the negative is cut into quarters, each quarter has only one-fourth the image, and so on. If the film were to be cut into a million pieces, each segment would have one-millionth of the image. Not so with the holographic negative. If the negative is cut into two halves, each half contains the entire image pattern and so can be reconstituted to form a whole image in space. If the holographic negative is cut into quarters, each quarter contains the entire image pattern and therefore can reproduce the whole object, and so on. Theoretically, if the holographic negative were cut into a million pieces, each portion would contain the whole of the original pattern, because the holographic plate or film is impregnated in such a way that every portion of the holographic negative "sees" the entire wave pattern.

So we jump to a key insight: I believe it possible that human consciousness is somehow analogous to the holographic plate and that each of us, representing a portion of this holographic negative, actually contains the total information of all consciousness past, present and future. The totality of this concept cannot be conceived three-dimensionally but must involve at least fourth-dimensional levels to be appreciated. In essence, this hypothesis states that each of us is part of a vast, totally aware state of consciousness and that each has access to that total awareness, limited only by our ability to conceive of it and by the modifications of the physical apparatus of conception itself.

This model can make understandable the ability of clairvoyants to see an action occurring at a distance, in the past, present or future. The clairvoyants don't go to that point in space. That point in space exists in their own consciousness, and, therefore, all they do is to observe the portion of their own consciousness that contains that segment going on elsewhere.

The same would be true of telepathy. If our own individual holographic negative contains the totality of awareness, we can have access to anybody's thought—past, present or future.

I believe this hypothesis is exactly true in all experiences, whether of the ordinary or superordinary kind. It is one way to explain how, often, several people will almost simultaneously create the same invention or have the same insight. It is consistent with both the mystical and the scientific statements that any action going on anywhere in the universe influences all points in the universe. Concepts of space are currently being completely restructured by theoretical physicists, and science now conceives that it is possible for an action at a distance to influence all points in space simultaneously, without any forces traveling through space. (There are some really excellent publications on this concept; one I particularly enjoy is *Space-Time and Beyond* by Bob Toben, with technical assistance from physicists Jack Sarfatti and Fred Wolf.)

I think the holographic model is an astonishing breakthrough in the comprehension of experiences in life. What fascinates me is the similarity between holographic images, projected into space, and the actual physical manifestations that one brings forth in space while in an altered state, such as instantaneous healing and so on. If you are similarly interested, you may wish to investigate current work on the theory of holographic solids and the developing techniques to form solid objects in vacant space. For more information I suggest *Scientific American*'s exceptionally clear presentations on holography over the last ten or twelve years.

I believe that reaching higher — or expanded, or natural — states of consciousness is merely the attuning of our central nervous system to perceptive states that have always existed in us but have been blocked by our outer mental conditioning and by our dwelling on our physical, emotional and sexual aspects.

The experiential awakening into expanded awareness is the hallmark of the Aquarian Age now commencing. Just as human consciousness is now distinguished from animal consciousness, the higher states of consciousness will differentiate the human beings who experience them from the ones who do not. While this experience at present is confined to relatively few people, I believe that those few foreshadow the future and that the quantum leap to higher consciousness will be experienced eventually by the entire human race.

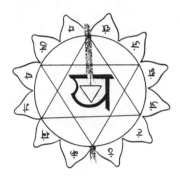

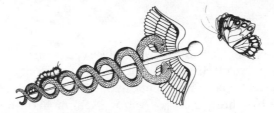

CHAPTER THREE

Energy, Experiments, Observers, Natural Teachers and the Three Injunctions

*Why must humans be trained into
natural states of consciousness? Because we have
chosen to believe in
illusion as the basis of reality.*

As I have already said, all experiences have the potential of teaching us about ourselves and about life. All is energy interaction, and all matter is energy, whether that matter be the billions of atoms that interact in forming a single cell, the inconceivable number of atoms that make up our physical bodies or the countless subatomic events that are our psyches. Nothing in the physical or psychological realm can become manifest unless energy in some form interacts with other energy, either in another or in a similar form. No event can take place unless something acts in relationship to something else.

In the past, science relied on observation as the means to derive data on which hypotheses and, eventually, theories of physical phenomena could be based. Today science is undergoing a reluctant but necessary shift in its approach. Now we are beginning to understand that the observer influences what is observed, just as the event observed influences the observer. Quantum mechanics and the theory of relativity predict this very concept. Old-time "controlled" experiments never considered the possibility that observation itself might influence the experiment, and as a result much of their data must be considered questionable today.

Some Soviet experiments—which we know only from unfortunately unclear translations—seem to indicate that the eyes of the observer emit a force field that can influence what the eyes are looking at. These studies are performed by placing petri dishes containing yeast before persons with open eyes and before others with closed eyes and noting differences in the growth of the two sets of cultures. Open eyes increase yeast growth. More important, it is reported that the energy from the eyes is measurable and that some observers have a greater intensity of emission than others.

Marcel Vogel, a researcher in California, has conducted experiments on highly concentrated solutions just before the chemicals in them are ready to crystallize. While observing these solutions under a microscope, he has found that he can influence the formation and the structure of such crystals by thought alone. Vogel's work may mean not only that we tend to see what we want to see through our own distorting filters, but also that we can influence what occurs simply by seeing it in our own way.

Many controlled studies cannot be reproduced by later experimenters not just because the work is influenced by some unidentified experimental factor (such as the altitude of the research center or slight variations in temperature) but because the person organizing the experiment actually may influence the results of the study in a way unsuspected by most scientists—and by that person. The psychological and physical fields that surround the researcher may be altering the results.

The force field of the human body, which parapsychology terms the "aura," extends from inches to many feet out from the body, depending upon the individual. Persons with clairvoyant vision see that auras interact with all matter in a given space. Similarly, Kirlian photography reveals that a person does have some form of biophysical energy emission of the body which can react with another person's biophysical energy. When two people place their index fingers on the same photographic plate, the interaction of their fields can be recorded with a motion picture camera.

In a somewhat similar, but significantly different, arrangement, the Kilner screen at the de la Warr Laboratory in London, England, uses a diocene dye between plates of glass to allow observers to watch what may be the auric fields of objects and people in interaction.

Although personal force fields are only now coming under the scrutiny of science, it should be emphasized that fields of energy have been observed for thousands of years by clairvoyants, and that average people, with training, can see or feel the grosser ones. Science is now beginning to confirm that auras and auric colors as seen by clairvoyant vision are fact. Science is also offering testing modalities to screen out people who feign these abilities.

Instrumentation developed by Valerie Hunt, Ph.D., of UCLA not only demonstrates the very high frequencies sometimes emitted from certain people's bodies but also correlates these very high energy frequencies with the auric colors seen by two independently tested clairvoyants, Rosalyn Bruyere and Carolyn Conger.

If all this energy radiation were just an interesting light show, I wouldn't bother to write about it. These energy fields, however, are involved in many interesting phenomena—in healing by the laying on of hands, in seeing and/or feeling abnormal energy fields emanating from the body or parts of the body of a person who is ill and in Uri Geller's ability not only to bend metallic objects, but to repair broken watches without touching them physically. The study of energy fields can also help us to understand the phenomenon of the Kundalini energy experientially explored by Tantric yogis in the East and in the West.

Above all, we must recognize that human consciousness is

capable of performance beyond our wildest imagination. Even though, for the verification of data, science prefers instruments and distrusts the mind, there never has been, nor will there ever be, an instrument superior to the mind, which creates instruments as extensions of itself.

Therefore, when I talk about the teaching experience of relating to any form in nature, I am not talking about just looking at it. I am talking about experiencing one's dynamic interaction with that object, about attempting to open oneself to subtler, vaster awarenesses.

During the first day of a two-week Conference at the ranch, I ask all the participants to spend the next several days seeking a teacher from the natural environment. They are simply to go out and try to experience what such a teaching form might reveal to them. I ask those persons who are particularly attuned to plants to seek a teacher in the mineral kingdom—a large rock, for instance—specifically to get out of their own "field" of sensitivity. I suggest that each individual, rather than just observing the desert, attempt to *become* the desert—an unbelievably deepening experience if one is able to release ego boundaries. But there is one catch in this task of finding a teacher from nature: the participants must allow the teacher to select them! They are warned that sometimes a teacher is teaching them when they least suspect it and that insight into that teaching may not come until hours or days later.

The participants struggle for, and almost invariably achieve, a level of consciousness that can enter into a communing process with these teachers. It is the struggle as much as the achievement that is so helpful in enabling humans to break out of their life-long patterns of feeling separated from the natural physical world and to realize that the human body is but one of many expressions of Life force.

The relationship with these teachers lasts the entire two weeks of the Conference. Before it is over, most participants will have spent several hours each day with their teacher— meditating, contemplating, touching, tasting, smelling, working with feeling tones and practicing the witnessing of their psychological reactions to the task.

The inspiration for this practice came from my own experience only a month after I left the world of science and medicine. I leased a house in the small village of Findhorn, Scotland, about a mile away from the now-famous Findhorn spiritual community, and in that setting I was amazed to find out how out of contact with the natural world I was. An animal was just an animal, and a tree was just a tree; I felt no relationship. But then, along the walk between my house and the Findhorn community, my consciousness was drawn to one of several magnificent pines growing in a grove. This particular tree seemed to be inviting me to embrace it. As I did so, I felt a charge pass through my body and a deep emotional response of loving and caring. As I wrote to a few friends — carefully selected ones, to be sure — I was having the most ridiculous love affair with a tree. Something within my physical body was capable of a relationship with a life form that still seemed alien to my confused outer mind. My body knew what it was doing, even if my mind didn't. The intellectual barriers began to crack as I experienced, for the first time in my adult life, the feeling of being part of the physical world.

Even to this day, I have to remind myself that I am a human being with a physical body beautifully similar to other life forms on the planet. All too often, I find myself living in my head, totally unaware of my form nature. Even now I sometimes remind myself of the Jules Feiffer cartoon of a man talking contemptuously to his body. It is just lucky that he needs it to carry his head around, he says. Otherwise, he would get rid of it!

In her last writings, which I came across several months ago, my mother stressed the importance of communicating with all forms in the *manifest plane* to achieve oneness with God. She spoke of listening to the sounds of rocks, trees, stones, whispering insects and all forms of creation. My intellectual pursuits had completely closed me off from the memory of her discussing this aspect of life, the teachers in nature.

I selected Sky Hi Ranch in Lucerne Valley, California, to explore my relationship to the desert. It is an environment with which most people have little experience, but every person eventually has to confront the desert of his or her own consciousness. The physical desert is a good place to begin.

To the uninitiated, the desert appears to be an enormous amount of decomposing granite, huge rock piles, endless acres of sage brush and large expanses of browns and light oranges. Gradually, though, the subtlety and beauty of this desert space begin to emerge: the subtle colors, ever more clearly differentiated and more varied; the rhythms of the desert, slow and undulating, like a vast silent sea; the plant and animal life exclusive in their habits, some so small that one has to get down on hands and knees to appreciate them; the silence, a disturbing element to the city dweller; and, of course, the vastness—God! the vastness of the desert, with its even vaster nighttime sky, demanding that one come out of the prison cell of one's consciousness.

The 560-acre ranch is located about 4,000 feet above sea level between the high Mojave Desert and the San Bernardino Mountains in what biological scientists call a transition zone. The biological transition zone is important to my work because my work is in the transition zones of consciousness.

All of us at all times are in relationship to all that surrounds us, and we are influenced by it. For beginning work in higher consciousness, a space that is unpolluted psychically and physically cannot be just imagined—it must be experienced. To remove oneself from the city, if only for such a brief time as two weeks, provides at least some opportunity to be free from inundation by literally hundreds of thousands of entrepreneurs vying for one's attention and from all the other psychic litter of man and machine. In the eighteen months before I began writing this book, more than five hundred people were introduced to the fundamentals of higher consciousness at Sky Hi Ranch. In groups of sixteen to twenty-six people, usually for two weeks, they were separated from their daily environments, isolated on the ranch, with no access to newspapers, television, radio or telephones. This isolation from the outer world was a significant factor in the changes that took place in all the participants, and each of them achieved heightened states of consciousness, even if only briefly.

When I say that each person must, at one time or another, explore the desert of consciousness, I am talking about the same kind of fundamentally important experience that appears as trips into the desert in the Bible and in many other masterworks. It is not simply the literal, physical desert that must be confronted but the essence that the desert represents. The mainspring of this adventure is the shift from the constructed aspects of reality to a perspective of limitless potential. One has to stretch the senses, reaching deeply for hidden resources. Without the lush, mothering nourishment of fertile forests or the moodiness and magnificence of the rapidly changing seashore, the desert appears barren. But instead of being barren the desert is really subtle, and subtlety is the essence of my teaching there.

Consciousness loves contrast. It is through the contrast of experiences that we are most likely to see most clearly. I said previously that one of the ways to approach the heightening aspects of the beginner's mind is to hold memory in check and to learn to appreciate repetitions of experience as if each repetition were the initial encounter. Allowing contrasting experiences, or entering into them, is a simple technique to heighten awareness. The greater the contrast, the more likely is awareness to pay attention. What greater contrast to the usual life pattern of a Westerner than to enter the desert in solitude?

I am reminded of a statement, by the vice-chancellor of a university in England, that I heard at a scientific conference in April 1975. This man, with impeccable credentials and a wealth of knowledge, was lamenting what he felt to be an error in the educational system. "More than 90 percent of what I teach," he commented, "is of an informational nature; less than 10 percent is derived from direct life experience." I was shocked. So much of my education was information, and so very little was direct experience. This thought impelled me to learn about myself not just through information and ideas about me but through direct experience of myself. Gradually, and later with greater acceleration, I began to leave the citadel of my intellect for longer and longer periods of time, with less and less anxiety. This process is painful, because it requires the ability to be devastatingly honest with oneself. I say that one must be able to draw the honesty cards—to accept what is before one's awareness, without rationalization or defense, in order to see clearly what is. To do so one must remember three injunctions: make no comparisons, make no judgments and delete your need to understand.

The story of the injunctions demonstrates both their possible usefulness and the possible consequences of not following them. In November 1975, a woman who lived near Redlands, California, came to the ranch for a personal consultation with me. In going into the reasons for her visit, she said that she had for some time been reading Tarot cards psychically. She was so gifted in accurately bringing through the future aspects of any question a client asked that she soon found herself inundated by phone calls from all over the world. Her talent in this particular psi area had become available to her eighteen months before her visit with me.

Now she very much wanted to be free of her psychic gift. She was emotionally unprepared to handle seeing negative events occurring in the future. Even when she was not reading the Tarot cards, she often became aware of traumatic events that were about to take place from minutes to hours after she perceived them. She had been so shaken by these experiences that a few months before coming to the ranch, she had stopped doing readings and had embarked on a course of study in conventional psychology at a nearby university. Respectable credentials and conventional work were more important to her than a strange ability that was, to her outer mind, upsetting and abnormal.

After we were well into her session, she suddenly remembered an event that had taken place three years before. She had mentioned it to no one else because she considered it an insane experience. A voice had spoken to her. She remembered the words perfectly; but even after three years, at the time of our conversation, they held no meaning for her.

This event happened some eighteen months *before* the onset of her psi ability. It occurred dramatically, and she had had no preparation for it. She emphasized to me that until then she had been a perfectly normal human being, without any knowledge of paranormal experiences or even of meditation. She was "just a housewife."

That the event took place in this context is important. To another person, it might have been the fulfillment of long years of spiritual preparation, but that woman at that time had no idea that such spiritual development was desirable—or even possible.

The episode occurred one day at sunset while she was walking along the beach in Santa Monica, California. Glancing down, she noticed that, as each foot sank into the sand, an iridescent light would appear, coming from the sand. Within a few minutes her feet also took on the eerie iridescence. She tried in vain to make the light go away, and at the same time she was deeply fascinated by it. As its many colors intensified, she lifted her gaze to watch the waves breaking on the shoreline, and she saw that the strange light emanated from the waves, too, as they crested and broke. Suddenly *everything* radiated this light in a fantastic display of color.

The woman lost all sense of time and normal spatial relationships, and she realized a feeling of overwhelming well-beingness, as if she were in a state of bliss where she was one with everything and all was God. As the experience came to its climax, she heard a booming voice. It was unlike anything she had ever heard. She was frightened by it, and she was afraid that she was going insane. The voice slowly and repetitively said to her: "There are three injunctions for you. Pay attention to them. Make no comparisons; make no comparisons. Make no judgments; make no judgments. Delete your need to understand; delete your need to understand."

The experience then faded gradually as she returned to ordinary consciousness. She was filled with wonder and with

fear. Instead of realizing that she had touched cosmic awareness, she believed that she had experienced insanity.

All of you who are working so diligently on achieving
cosmic consciousness through long, and sometimes painful,
disciplined practices, take note! The event was spontaneous,
totally unexpected, fully developed and occurred in a woman to
whom, at least in this lifetime, its significance and nature were
completely veiled. It came *before* the development of her ability
to transcend the barriers of space and time. I stress these points,
because I strongly suspect that experiences of this nature occur
in ordinary people much more frequently than they are reported
and that what keeps these people silent is the fear of being
thought abnormal or psychotic.

"Make no comparisons." Time and time again we are
conditioned to evaluate ourselves in relationship to other people
through competitive examinations, sports, promotions, social
standing, and so on. Each society has its own selection of
criteria to which its people must measure up, by which they are
compared. If our particular psychological or physical makeup
does not meet the standard, we experience trauma. Yet we,
ourselves, are the ones who create this trauma, because it is not
the rejection or nonacceptance by other people but nonacceptance or rejection by ourselves that causes the pain.

The tendency to live in *ideas* about reality isolates the mind
from the true reality of the physical level. But the idea level has
an impossible time when it is directly confronted by the manifest level. Self *is* — the self is true, without question — but
ideas about self may be true or false, and in this ambiguity lies
the problem. If the individual insists on holding on to *ideas*
rather than harmonizing with *what is*, pain must follow. The
individual then is driven to take stronger defensive measures,
and repression, depression and abreaction (to name a few)
compound the difficulty. The ability to experience and to flow
with *what is* signals the beginning of the unification of mind,
body and spirit. It is the first initiation into a natural state of
Beingness.

Are we too fat, too short, too tall, too uneducated, too intellectual, too emotional, too feminine, too masculine, too strange, too undisciplined, too weak, too immature, too compulsive, too unspiritual, too ungifted? Do we criticize ourselves because we smoke or don't smoke? Because we drink or don't drink? Because we are religious or not religious? The list of possibilities is endless. Rooted in the injunction "Make no comparisons" is the corollary idea: be whatever you are. Experience of the self, not any preconceived ideas about the various aspects of the self, is what should dictate whether something should be changed.

In Conference work at the ranch, this injunction comes up repeatedly. As the first participants begin to experience expanded states of consciousness, the others, observing them, start the self-whipping process: they report that they feel left out, inadequate, insecure and relatively worthless. When I point out to them that they could be resonating with the experience the expanded member is enjoying, opening to the experience, and rejoicing in another's accomplishment, they begin to understand how their own minds obstruct expanded awareness, how they and their comparisons are holding back their own growth. Actually, the heightened individual helps to heighten others through the principle of *induction*. That is, the heightened person's level of consciousness is reflected in his or her body-energy field so that a similar response is induced in the second person's energy field, and that response moves on to the second person's awareness.

Induction works better if the second person's induction field isn't blocked by defenses. Unfortunately, the process of comparison is not the only cause of defenses. It often happens that, even though the aspirant's outer mind envisions the heightening experience as desirable, the individual feels threatened on some inner level by the fear of loss of control. To defend against that imagined loss, a reactive block is established.

Again I offer experience from my own life as an example. Through most of my life, I saw my body as less masculine in form than the ideal I held and the standard I was convinced others held. My right testicle was undescended until I was fourteen, I didn't need to shave until I was nineteen and my beard growth is patchy. Mild breast enlargement was noted in adolescence, my skin was too smooth and my relative lack of body hair, especially on the chest, was unacceptable to me. I believed that there was something wrong with me. It was not until I reached my early thirties that I realized the fallaciousness of this self-made trauma. I now have no need to compare myself to any other human form and certainly not to an image of a different self, one that doesn't even exist. When my self-rejection began to crumble, the energy that had gone into my psychological defenses was released into a deep sense of appreciation and wonderment at the infinite variations that form nature displays.

The comparison process literally locks us into a prison filled with psychological pain. Until I could reach a state of awareness that each individual is a distinct and unique representation of form and psyche, I was trapped. Then awareness let me out of the prison and led me to the astonishing truth: we are far more than we possibly could wish, but we are herded into a narrow spectrum of beliefs about who and what we are. To begin to awaken into this potential experience of our own individual wholeness demands that no comparisons be made. There is only one entity in the entire plane who can make the comparison that generates the vicious cycle, and that entity is you.

My greatest test of self-value came during the night of the full moon in February 1975 when I spent thirteen hours alone in the Great Pyramid of Cheops. One of many profound experiences that night was the presentation of every flaw of my Beingness, each one rapidly flashed before my awareness like a series of photographic slides in supervivid color and detail. Seeing them, I knew that I could choose between reacting and observing, and I chose the latter. The totality of my Beingness then flashed before me, and, with insight into each flaw, I no longer saw them as flaws, but rather, as challenges, necessary experiences for my unfolding and awakening.

There is a quotation from Goethe: "If you treat man as he appears to be, you make him worse than he is. But if you treat man as if he already were what he potentially could be, you make him what he should be." The key word is *appears*. Rarely, if ever, do we see the totality — including the potential not yet manifest — of ourselves or of another human being; the filtering system of the outer mind is too strong. In Conferences at the ranch, after I deliver the Goethe quotation to participants, I ask that each spend an entire afternoon paraphrasing this quotation into a contemplation of: "If I treat myself as I think I appear to be, I make myself less than I am. But if I treat myself as if I already were what I potentially could be, I make myself what I should be." Only linear, time-trapped thoughts prevent us from seeing the staggering beauty of our entirety.

Ideas about what is right and what is wrong are, in the vast majority of cases, not intrinsically valid. They can be valid only relative to the perspective of the consciousness that holds them; and, as we have seen, they can be mistaken even then. There are many, many value systems, as one can easily discern in traveling through the world; and each has its own ideas of right and wrong. The awakening process brings one to the deeper wisdoms wherein one finds a preference for that which feels harmonious, natural, uplifting, expanding and inspiring. Instead of striving for *ideas* of what ought to be, one chooses what fits into *what is*.

It is especially important that one not interpret the injunction against making comparisons as an exhortation to live in a state of complacency, where everything that the outer mind sees is rationalized as being perfect or right, without need for change. Complacency is the way of the ignorant. The critical key here is to unhook the emotional or psychological defense mechanisms so that one may begin to see and accept what is coming from more expanded states of awareness. What appears undesirable from a less inspired state may be in perfect harmony from a higher point of view.

We are all in different stages of development in awareness. The ever-expanding realizations that eventually bring one into illumination or mastery of one's current level of existence are a natural process in the experience of Life. Each of us chooses whether to honor that deeper yearning for spiritual fulfillment when it begins to emerge into awareness. The most common choice is to ignore it, to sink back into comfortable, established life patterns already conveniently rationalized as real and important.

If one is fundamentally content with one's life, if there is no strong suspicion that there is more to Beingness than what the usual human being calls life, if one does not feel a pull toward any other level of awareness, then there is no need to be reading a book discussing the Transformational Process. As I warned in the introduction, the moment one begins to seek the path for change and expansion of awareness, one's life changes, often dramatically. Once the nectar is tasted, there is no turning back. Like the outgrown clothing of youth, the old patterns and beliefs no longer fit. A sense of constriction and pain will be experienced if one tries to continue embracing one's old gods.

"Make no judgments." All judgments of the kind meant in this second injunction issue out of conditioned value systems, which in turn have roots in the emotional-reflex arc. A judgment of this kind can be only a reaction to what is experienced. Note the word *reaction* because it is the criterion to determine whether the response is a conditioned one and not an intrinsic value. Our reactions to good or bad, beautiful or ugly, talented or untalented are trained responses related to the culture and subculture of our upbringing and education. Before one commits oneself to a judgment, one must at least attempt to see whence the reaction came. If it is an idea also held by mother or father, a teacher, an authority figure in a religious institution, you must ask yourself whether it is a valid, natural response in its own right or whether it has been conditioned in you by those authorities. Do you have an alternative to the perspective from which you are viewing and experiencing the situation? The task is to discern an event, to see it clearly, at first without response.

Then one's later response is a clue to one's level of development or awakening. Human consciousness becomes rigid through training. Once it has been conditioned, it cannot appreciate natural states of experience without being retrained.

In Rudolf Steiner's book *Theosophy*, the last chapter, entitled "The Path of Knowledge," contains some profound words on the consequences of judgment:

> One of the first qualities that everyone wishing to acquire a vision of higher facts has to develop...is the unreserved, unprejudiced laying of oneself open to what is revealed by human life or by the world external to man....Knowledge is received only in those moments in which every judgment, every criticism coming from ourselves, is silent....Anyone who wishes to tread the path of higher knowledge must train himself to be able at any given moment to obliterate himself with all his prejudices. As long as he obliterates himself the revelations of the new world flow to him....This open-minded and uncritical laying of ourselves open has nothing to do with blind faith. The important thing is not that we should believe blindly in anything, but that we should not put a blind judgment in the place of the living impression.

"Delete your need to understand." Notice that this third and final injunction does not ask one to delete understanding. It clearly warns against hanging on to the *need* to understand, which stems from preconditioned areas of the psyche. Direct knowledge or understanding simply is, and it has nothing to do with need on the part of the observer. The *need* to understand comes between the observer and what is being presented to the awareness. It hinders, gets in the way. The need to understand indicates a need to control, to live by the idea rather than flowing with the reality of higher consciousness. Let go of the

need to understand, just as you let go of comparisons and judgments, so that you can experience, without encumbrances, what really is.

As for the woman who heard the voice on the beach, what she related was obviously an experience in cosmic awareness. If she had understood and followed the three injunctions she received, she might never have had to experience pain from what came into her life by way of her breakthrough into higher dimensions of consciousness. All three injunctions have to do with giving up ideas of what ought to be and accepting what is, and it is from hanging on to what ought to be and rejecting what is that pain comes.

And, let me add, even as great a psychic gift as hers is only one of many initial experiences in spiritual-psychological development.

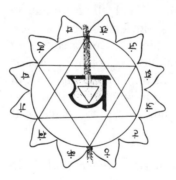

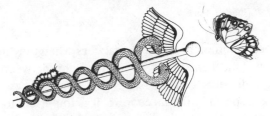

CHAPTER FOUR

Dream Analysis, Telepathy, the Tarot and the *I Ching*

"But my eyes have seen the Glory,"
I protested. "Go deeper," the Inner Teacher replied.

"What meaning does a teacher — any kind of teacher — impart to me concerning my perspective and my exploration?" As one goes deeper into the Transformational Process, that question is to be kept in the forefront of one's awareness, because the discovery of the mechanisms of one's own mind begins during this phase of observing the relationships of external events to changing internal perspectives.

Teachers are only scaffoldings on which experiences display themselves. It is the experience of life, not the scaffolding of life, that we wish to examine in detail. For this purpose a working knowledge of dream analysis, the Tarot and the *I Ching* is invaluable in accelerating the expansion of awareness. These teaching forms are scaffoldings — or instruments, vehicles, or tools, if you prefer — that offer the opportunity to integrate into the experience of the self that which at first seems to be other than or external to the self. Telepathy is an exper-

67

ience common to all these teachers when they are perceived as deeper mechanisms of communication between the aspects of the individual consciousness.

Especially in this context, it is important to realize that the word "external" is relative. Although many experiences in conscious awareness are usually considered external to the self, all experiences actually originate within the individual's consciousness. It is not hard to see the truth of this statement in the case of dreams, the filtered interpretation of the Tarot cards or the filtered interpretation of what a human teacher teaches, but it also includes any impression of the external world on the cortex of the brain. Most people, most of the time, consider these experiences to be not their own but somehow to originate outside themselves, to be external. Actually, the initial areas on which some teachers focus are the psychological mechanisms that block the full flow of external stimuli, whether of light, sound, other electromagnetic waves or even wave forms not yet discovered or defined. Teachers try to help make the external, internal.

Many volumes, both profound and superficial, have been written on dreams and their interpretation, as well as on the Tarot and on the study of psychological defense mechanisms. It is not my intention to give an in-depth discussion of these areas, but rather to concentrate on what I have found most useful in the understanding of the two states of ordinary human awareness, the conscious and the unconscious.

I have often asked myself: how did human beings get into such a farcical state of Beingness as to have the vaster portion of their consciousness relegated to an unaware, seemingly fathomless pit? How is it that, so to speak, the right hand doesn't know what the left hand is doing? To extend this analogy: does the left hand (the unconscious) know everything, including what the right hand is doing, while the right hand (the conscious) only knows what it, itself, is doing — and that only sometimes? Have we become identified with only a small segment of our potential awareness, forgetting or deliberately excluding the remainder? It is evident that we have, and when I get to the chapter on body-energy fields, it will be even more evident that we have excluded the vaster, more significant areas not only of our awareness but of our physical Beingness as well.

The veil between the aware and the unaware states of consciousness is one focus of my current study. We don't need to *develop* higher states of consciousness, because they already exist within us. What we need is to break down the artificial partitions that keep us from experiencing total awareness. When we start to understand how the mind operates at the ordinary levels, we have at least the beginning approach to rending this veil. At that point the ushering in of a unified state of consciousness has begun. Then the challenge is to accelerate the process.

According to the generous statistics of psychologists, we are about 20 percent aware and 80 percent unaware of our actions and motivations. I would suggest, more realistically, that we are less than 0.0001 percent awake and more than 99.9999 percent unconscious. The psychologists arrived at less embarassing figures because they did not acknowledge the multidimensional aspects of human awareness beyond the everyday outer mind. The appalling extent of our usual unconscious can be appreciated — excruciatingly — only when one has experienced expanded, mystical, cosmic or, in my term, the natural, unpartitioned states of awareness. One does not know how limited the ordinary awareness is until it is contrasted against a more expanded one.

I really enjoy encountering die-hard rationalists who dismiss expanded experiences not just as fantasy but, even more extremely, as nonexistent — and I meet such people often. Not only do they want proof (of which there is plenty), but they demand proof that fits the structure of their beliefs about the physical world. To them the simple truth is that, since they haven't experienced expanded consciousness, it doesn't — perhaps cannot — exist. When these skeptics begin to come into expanded awareness, I cannot help but laugh. They are overwhelmed, slightly disoriented and sometimes enraged that they could have been so ignorant in such a recent past. No words are needed: the experience suffices. From the expanded state, the so-called real world appears to be a crazy patchwork quilt, a shambles of disorganized reality and, of course, only partial reality at that. From expanded awareness, the return to ordinary perception is like returning to a very retarded human's state of mind.

The emphasis in my work is to bring expanded states of awareness to the experiential level of individuals, first by sharing a conceptual framework, then by demonstrating the mechanisms of consciousness that block the experiences and finally through the example of my own Beingness. This sharing, this demonstration and this example consistently bring about the direct experience, for which no words, profound or simple, can even be an adequate substitute.

As I have recognized only in the last year, the mere presence of a being who enjoys periods of natural awareness can be very important in this process. In fact, I am now certain that absolutely no dialogue or action is necessary for individuals to be heightened into expanded awareness when they are in the presence of such a teacher. In a way unconscious to the seeker's awareness, the seeker's energy field is freed from its old patterns and reshapes itself on the energy field of the teacher. Then the nonordinary simply begins to be experienced. The words, the teaching sessions, the exercises are only scaffoldings that hold the individual's attention long enough for this process of induction to occur. The teacher, as long as he or she is operating in expanded awareness, could talk about anything at all, and still achieve the same results.

The teacher's voice vibration can augment the experience, but, to repeat, it is not the words or their content that cause the change. It is the sound, which could as well be made in gibberish or in chanting. Words and their content may expand the abstract intellectual portion of consciousness, but ideas alone do not and cannot cause induction. The control and mastery of sound waves is part of the path of a teacher. If you have read Frank Herbert's *Dune* novels, you may already have some idea of voice vibration and its power.

In the movement from the divided to the unified state of

awareness, the concept of the central room might be helpful. In March 1975, I was in meditation at Auroville — an international, interracial, spiritual commune, under the aegis of the now-deceased Sri Aurobindo, that was located on the southeastern coast of India, near the old French town of Pondicherry. During meditation, I was struck by an image of a large, central room on the second floor of a three-storied, many-roomed mansion. I saw myself seated in this central room that was brilliantly lighted from a source above my head. From this central position, I didn't have to get up to enter one room and then another or to go upstairs or downstairs to observe what was happening in the structure, because the building was made of transparent crystal. The image reverberated through me and became an insight: there is such an observational state of consciousness inside my own awareness!

Conceiving the possibility enabled me to begin the experience. The next step was to break down the logical linear perspective and thus to conceive that natural awareness does not have to concentrate on only one thing at a time. In the central room, more and more events can be experienced — simultaneously. Although I have not yet mastered it completely, the phenomenon of multiple perspectives is developing rapidly in my awareness.

This anecdote contains the significant initial insights that can begin to unify a divided or partitioned consciousness. It serves as a model for observing not only the subconscious activity (the ground level of the envisioned mansion), but the superconscious aspects, as well (the third-story level). The second level has many other chambers in addition to the central room — exactly as in sequestered ordinary awareness. The ability to see clearly is only the beginning. Eventually, the crystal partitions are transmuted, and unification is complete.

Linear outer communication reflects the partitions of the outer mind. If I ask people to relate their problem to me, they begin to verbalize first one idea and then another — in linear outer communication — until they feel that the problem has been described. While they are doing so, I close my eyes and attempt to image the impression of the total situation, using their words to guide me to the level and area of their consciousness where the conflict has configurated itself. This technique uses a form of telepathic rapport.

It was a long time before I first encountered a client who used telepathy consciously, who understood that the totality of any given problem or awareness could be instantaneously transmitted. Then I met Carolyn Conger. I knew before I met her that she was clairvoyant, but I did not suspect the degree of development in all the psi areas. Naively, I began our session together by asking her to tell me her problems. I closed my eyes, awaiting the words that would carry me to the area of her consciousness where the problem was. After waiting a full five minutes for her to begin talking, I suspected that the problem must be so emotionally charged that she could not express herself. Finally I told her to start just anywhere and the words would come. She burst out laughing and only then began to tell the reasons for coming to see me.

A year later, when I knew her better, she told me what had occurred during the first five minutes of that consultation, and by then I, too, found it quite humorous. She had already picked up that I was capable of telepathic rapport, and so she began the session by flashing the totality of her problem to me telepathically. I, however, had put myself into a set to receive feeling tones and not images. I had no idea what was going on. The tables had been turned, and I didn't even know it. So that she would not embarrass me, Carolyn had finally resorted to words when I, with great compassion, had urged her to begin.

In July 1977, Carolyn and I started work together on direct-image telepathy, an experience far more exciting than feeling-tone telepathy. We began by setting aside time in the morning while we were eating breakfast. I would start by drawing something on a piece of paper — a stick figure, a geometric design, a bird, whatever — and then would create a feeling to associate with it. When I had both aspects well in mind, I would signal that I was ready, and Carolyn would tell me what her impression was. This procedure was particularly easy for her, and she missed little — even when I mixed a negative feeling state with a positive or happy drawing. The addition of a feeling state somehow helps to intensify what is telepathically impressed and so is very helpful for the beginner at receiving. When it was her turn to impress my awareness with her drawing and her feeling-tone, I would concentrate on picking up the feeling. At first, greater intensity of her feeling — anger, frustration, or whatever — made it easier for me to tell what the feeling was; later I could receive less intense feelings telepathically. After I had an impress of the feeling, I would wait until an image appeared in my mind. Sometimes it was very clear, but most of the time it was indistinct. Occasionally I would see no image but the word for the image would pop into my mind. At other times I would be talking about the feeling-tone I was sensing when I would suddenly shift and say what object she was using.

As Carolyn says, "It's just like thinking. An idea just emerges into your awareness.... How an idea appears in consciousness is unknown, and neither is the way a telepathic impress appears.... The more you can relax and allow the phenomenon, the more accurate the results." What Carolyn stresses is that one doesn't send or receive anything: in the state of awareness where telepathic impressions are experienced, the sender and the receiver are one and the same person. It is another example of the hologram principle. I can easily impress to Carolyn, whether she is in the same room or miles away, but so far I am only sporadically able to sense her images. This work is inspiring to me, because it foreshadows what human beings in general will be experiencing within the next one hundred years. Words are unsatisfactory when direct-image and feeling-tone telepathies have been experienced.

Once again, it is acculturation that selects and conditions only a few of the many possible aspects of awareness. In our Western, material, technological culture, the primary emphasis is on the intellectual, the idea abstractions, to the almost total exclusion of simultaneous or multidimensional states of consciousness. Sexuality and emotive responses are similarly conditioned into limited patterns. Sequential linear awareness is an important and useful tool in its place, but it certainly is not the culmination of awareness, and it will eventually be revalued: instead of being dominant, as it is today, it will become the instrument of a higher organizer or orchestrator of consciousness. This higher orchestrator will represent the central room in the crystal mansion, the unified state of Beingness.

Why do I discuss Carolyn Conger and telepathy in a section on dreams? Because dreams are direct-image communications: one portion of our consciousness impresses itself telepathically on another part. We will discover as we go on that telepathy is not just one means of communication but is probably the basic mechanism of all thought.

In the West, the works of Sigmund Freud and of Carl Jung made the initial breakthroughs into the subconscious. The East has been hundreds, if not thousands, of years ahead of the West in the awareness of subconscious and superconscious states but has been vastly limited in practice by restrictions on the kinds and numbers of people who were allowed to learn this information. The Western mystery schools and various occult schools, from pre-Egyptian times onward, transmitted forth the teachings of higher states of consciousness but, again, conveyed them only to a very few. Only in the past one hundred years have the deeper esoteric wisdoms been brought forth to the public in the West. The amplification of this trend over the past ten years is astounding.

The ancients enjoined us against revealing the secret teachings to the masses for fear of misuse of the powers they engender. In my experience this fear is ungrounded, because even when you reveal ancient techniques or knowledge gleaned over many lifetimes, few can understand them, and even fewer can make use of them. By the time a soul reaches the state of consciousness in which to use and to develop further such gifts, he or she is aware of the action-reaction law, the law of Karma: no one escapes the consequences of misuse of power, whether it be temporal material power or powers not yet conceived by the general public.

For millenia, Eastern teachers have propagated the idea that the psychic levels concerned with manipulation of the physical plane are to be shunned, excluded from experience, because they represent less than the supreme state that can be reached and the danger of being caught in power and glamour is too great. I find this kind of teaching ironic, because every soul has to work through personal power in his or her development on the way to that supreme state. If our task is to become totally aware — which I believe is the evolutionary sequence of each soul — the idea of excluding the higher natural states of awareness is inconceivable. There is validity in the concern that a person's development will be retarded if the soul becomes trapped in the psychic awareness; but instead of avoiding any stage of the journey, the way onward is to experience any and all states without clutching them, to allow the adventure in awareness to unfold without grasping or trying to retain any part of it. On the other hand, one must not will the manifestation of psychic states prematurely. These energies can heal or destroy, send one to the heights or plunge one into the depths — as souls who are power-driven know well. I spent the greater part of the first thirty-five years of this lifetime working through personal power, and I still have not finished resolving its subtler areas.

Up through the years when I was in medical school, the autonomic nervous system — which controls all the body's involuntary functions, such as the tonus of the vascular system; the heart rate; smooth muscles' activity in the respiratory, digestive and excretory systems; and so on — was thought to be strictly outside the control of the conscious mind. In Western science biofeedback was the first major breakthrough to demonstrate the fallacy of this belief. In the East, the conscious control of the autonomic nervous system, achieved without instruments, has been a feat well-known to yogis and high lamas for centuries. Volitional control over brain-wave patterns — and, by implication, volitional control over altered states of consciousness — is an additional technique developed by Western technology and, again, is a replication of much earlier explorations by the Eastern mystics and occultists. (Excellent books on biofeedback, notably those by Barbara Brown, are available.) But biofeedback is only one approach that is currently opening the veil between the unaware and aware portions of consciousness.

Dream analysis is the "royal road" into a portion of the unconscious psyche, but it is severely limited by the skill of the interpreter and by the ability of the client to remember the dream.

Eunice Hurt, my second teacher, placed great emphasis on dream interpretation. Fortunately for her work, her psi abilities enabled her to recall the details of a dream told to her, even when the dreamer did not remember them! She could literally dream the dream of the dreamer, but she did not have to go to sleep to do it. In this section, I wish to relate some of the techniques she shared, along with those I have developed in the six years since her death.

Certain basic principles underlie my current hypothesis regarding dream work. These ground rules have proved invaluable in gaining insight into both myself and others. It will become apparent that I am not a traditional dream analyst, psychiatric or otherwise, nor have I been formally trained in the art. It simply comes naturally to me.

1. First and foremost, dreams are as valid conscious realities as the reality experienced in the outer awake state. I am using the word *awake* in its generally accepted sense, because, as I have already implied, I consider the outer awake state quite sleepy (retarded), if not asleep (comatose). The fact that a dream may make no rational sense to the outer mind does not justify disregarding it. Like a foreign language, its organization and form of communication must be learned. A person speaking Tibetan could be showering forth the pearls of the ages, but the message would be totally lost to the listener untrained in the language. So it is with dreams and their messages.

2. Unlike the outer mind, the subconscious and superconscious areas are not limited in their range of experiences and forms of communication, nor are these areas identified with a

particular body, belief system or the construct called time. They do not have to distinguish between self and other-than-self, and physical laws are of no concern to them.

3. Dream realities are far closer to our natural states of Beingness than even the most highly intensified outer reality. To my mind, dreams demonstrate conclusively that general human consciousness is not composed of unique, isolated, self-initiated units that can learn only through outer teachers. Indeed, the individual consciousness is part of a vast collective pool of total human awareness, the collective unconscious. When the outer mind is blocked by social conditioning, the dream reality can tap the collective unconscious and communicate it to the outer mind. Later, when the outer awareness is able to tap the same collective pool volitionally, the state of initial illumination is reached and the dream function diminishes, because it is no longer needed as much as before.

4. Clearly, the dream state is not the unconscious but is an intermediate state between the aware and the unaware, a mechanism that has some of the qualities of both states. True dreaming states are under the primary direction of the unconscious; while the waking dream states, such as fantasy, are primarily influenced by the outer mind.

5. In true dreaming states, the consciousness of the individual witnessing the dream cannot know that it is dreaming. All that is experienced is absolutely (in the relative sense) real to the experiencing awareness. This is a key point to emphasize, because it enables the comprehension that our total Beingness is multidimensional, participating simultaneously in many reality systems. Only the focus of awareness determines which reality dimension or state of consciousness is perceived as real.

6. Ramana Maharshi, an East Indian saint, made a salient point: the observer who witnesses the outer reality state is the same observer who witnesses the dream reality states. There is no true distinction between the two or more states of Beingness. Keep in mind that, while you are in the inner dream state nothing is going to convince you that the reality experienced there is not valid—just as when you are in the normal awake

state nothing is going to convince you that it, too, isn't the real reality. The task is to know yourself as the observer of both states.

7. The outer awake state is as much a dream as the inner dream state is a reality. All the techniques used to interpret dream states can be employed to interpret the outer dream. At this level of awareness, the unconscious activity common to both the inner and the outer dream states can be clearly seen, because the same dynamics occur in both. Jungian analysts, who are relatively developed in inner dream interpretation, fail to take this crucial step in working with clients, and it is a severe limitation in their work, as it is in any other psychoanalytic process that employs dream analysis. It is such a simple step to take. All one has to do is to ask the client to describe the preceding day's activities and analyze this report as if it were a dream. Contained within the narration of the outer dream will be all the clues one usually uncovers when analyzing inner dreams. Just as in the inner dream state, unconscious patterns operate in the awake state and influence all action and all perception of that action. As in the inner dream, the individual is unconscious of the patterns displayed. The success of this approach has been demonstrated both in my individual consultations and in group Conference work.

8. If we concede that all realities are varieties of dream states — an insight thousands of years old — and that there are dreams within dreams within dreams, the next concept can be considered. In the analyst-client interaction, there are at least five different dreams that come from the beginning in the dreamer's consciousness:

(1) The original dream of the dreamer
(2) The dream as related by the dreamer
(3) The dream that appears in the mind of the analyst as the dreamer relates the dream
(4) The dream that appears in the mind of the dreamer as the analyst interprets the related dream
(5) The dream that appears in the mind of the analyst as the dreamer interprets his or her own dream

Eunice Hurt was the only person I ever met who could directly experience the dream of the dreamer. The usual analyst is dealing almost exclusively with secondary or tertiary dream states, primarily the latter. These dream states may not be anything like the original dream, but they can give enough insight into the dreamer's consciousness to be of value. In the initial phases of dream work, the analyst is, in fact, interpreting his or her own dream (the third) and not that of the dreamer. As the analyst becomes more self-aware, there is less and less of this distortion. The best dream work allows both client and analyst to see each other's dynamics through the mutual interpretation of the four dreams after the original one.

The retelling of the dream always changes it. The changes that are made are significant, because they reveal further unconscious dynamics. I know of only two people who can interpret another person's dream, as retold, without distorting the information they hear from the dreamer. A great deal of information can be gleaned about the psychodynamics of analysts from the ways they interpret dreams and from the selection of parts they stress. The same is true, of course, of the dreamer who is interpreting the original dream.

The dreamer must always be the first to analyze, or to try to analyze, the original dream. If the analyst interprets the dream before the dreamer struggles through his or her own interpretation, no matter how inept it may be, the dreamer remains ignorant of the actual practice of dream analysis and remains tied to the analyst. In addition, the analyst loses the opportunity to observe the dreamer's defenses as they distort or cause forgetting in the dreamer's interpretation. These dynamics are well-known to the dream analyst but rarely known to the dreamer. When the client cannot participate fully, the analyst also loses the opportunity to develop his or her own self-awareness.

Most therapists in any field of psychology or psychiatry do not like to expose their own unconscious dynamics. I strongly disagree with this attitude. Mutual exploration is a far better teaching interaction than the usual student-teacher interaction or the client-professional interaction. Holistic medicine has the magnificent attribute of breaking down the professional barrier so that the physician and the patient explore the problems as cohorts instead of perpetuating the old, false dichotomy between the all-knowing (the professional or the teacher) and the ignorant (the client or student). In the best of holistic exchanges, mystiques and myths are shattered. Each of the interacting human beings is sharing openly and honestly.

For the client, the important goal of dream interpretation is not the understanding of this or that dream but the power to achieve self-insight, the ability to carry out dream interpretation independently in the future. For this reason I have sometimes had people work on the interpretation of individual dreams for days, weeks or even months while I withheld my own insights. If I withhold or do not deliver my insights to them first, they are sometimes appalled, sometimes angered, sometimes frightened and most certainly frustrated; but when they experience insight into a dream on their own, no words, no amount of money, no external gift could possibly be equivalent to the reward of self-realization they experience. No healer helps his or her clients by doing for them what they can do for themselves.

9. As skill in dream interpretation increases, group sharing of dreams can be an amazing accelerator of individual self-realization. One person's primary dream may generate many #2, #3, #4 and #5 dreams in other people in the group. As they observe the unconscious dynamics of their fellows, participants more readily grasp their own unconscious dynamics. Out of a group of twenty people, nineteen may be blocked from seeing the unconscious pattern at work in a particular dream; the clear perception of the twentieth person may be enough to release them all.

10. Because dreams are mosaics, the first important step in the interpretation of a dream is to record every detail accurately, no matter how insignificant or absurd it may seem. Dream journals are invaluable. A notebook or tape recorder by the bedside can be very helpful, because it is often difficult to keep the focus of awareness in the dream reality long enough to record it. (At first many of my dreams were lost because I was

absolutely sure that I would remember the dream next morning, only to have it evaporate upon arising.) There is also a meditative technique for recapturing dreams that I'll discuss when I cover state-bound consciousness.

11. At least in the initial phases of dream work, the specific details of a dream are important only insofar as they guide the analysis to the general pattern or patterns displayed. As is well-known to traditional dream analysts, each component of a dream is symbolic of an aspect of the dreamer's consciousness, whether it involves people, places, events, moods, actions or things. Nothing in a dream is superfluous, but initially little if any of it is to be taken literally. Insights lie in discovering the essence of the symbols.

12. There is never an absolute interpretation of any dream symbol. Both inner dreams and outer dreams are multidimensional, with many levels of meaning all simultaneously interacting. An object in one dream may appear in another dream and have an entirely different symbolic essence. This aspect of dream interpretation, so very difficult to teach, represents the mastery of the art of dream analysis, as distinguished from a cookbook approach to dream symbols. A body of water in a dream may mean the unconscious, the spiritual, the feminine, fluidity, urine, the emotions, movement from one place to another, a need fulfilled or a multiplicity of other things. The pattern and relationship of objects and events helps guide one into a relatively functional interpretation. The best dream analysts are intuitive, and so are the best dream analyses.

13. The way a dream is lighted appears to be significant. In my experience, dreams that are brilliantly colored and super-vivid reflect the superconscious state and are always deeply meaningful to the dreamer. If such a dream comes through, don't lose it. In my own life, these dreams are invariably prophetic. Except in those persons who invariably dream in color, dreams of usual color intensity are from the mental or higher creative areas of consciousness. Dreams in subdued lighting — shadowy, with a dark greenish or brownish tone, or in black and white — are from the emotional-astral levels.

Dreams of even darker quality are from deep subconscious areas.

14. I find it extremely valuable to interpret each aspect of my own dreams from seven different perspectives:

(1) Literal physical perspective
(2) Sexual perspective
(3) Emotional perspective
(4) Collective human perspective
(5) Higher creative perspective
(6) Mental intellectual perspective
(7) Universal perspective, which synthesizes the other six perspectives

In general a specific dream will appear to be, as a whole, centered in one of the seven groupings, while its component parts may reflect either the same level or others. The level of the dream as a whole gives a good indication of which unconscious area is unresolved in the dreamer.

15. An interesting phenomenon occurs in dream interpretation — what I call the "zing" — a feeling sensation in the awareness of both the analyst and the dreamer when the interpretation is precisely in tune with what the dream was communicating.

16. In analyzing dreams, it is essential to remember the three injunctions from the last chapter. *Make no comparisons. Make no judgments. Delete the need to understand.* Psychological sets and emotional reactions make it impossible to analyze dreams.

17. Another technique I have found helpful in working on my own dreams is to tell my dream to someone else and have him or her relate it back to me as if it were his or her dream. Seeing it as another person's dream will often unblock my consciousness long enough for me to get the insight.

There are two other aspects of dream work worth mentioning. The first is that there are rare people who can literally dream a dream *for* another person. (This process is not the same as

Eunice's apparently unique ability. She could recover your dream telepathically after you had already dreamed it. These other unusual persons can take your place and dream a dream that you have never dreamed but that is entirely yours.) This art has been known since ancient times. In the healing temples of ancient Greece, a seeker of prophetic advice would consult a priestess gifted in this art; the priestess would then enter a natural state of sleep; and upon awakening, she would report to the seeker what she had experienced. Drugs and trance states were used in the same way.

A woman psychiatrist in Los Angeles has told me several dreams she has had about me. In each case she had the sensation that the dream did not belong to her. She has also had other dreams involving me but sensed these dreams as her own. When she reports one of "my" dreams to me, I immediately recognize the significance to me and can in no way interpret it as if it belonged to her.

The second aspect of dream work I am beginning to explore is the potential of a dream experienced in common by several members of a group at the same time. Each member of the group is to ask his or her own consciousness to be open to experiencing a community dream. No other specific suggestion is made. After retiring they are to implant this suggestion in their minds during twilight sleep, the hypnagogic state on the border between sleep and wakefulness. So far, individuals have reported dreams involving the group, but never have two or more people reported a similar dream from the same night. I do believe a group dream to be possible, however, and I think that the participants at this time are not yet sufficiently unified in group consciousness to experience the phenomenon. The initial two-week Conferences emphasize self-realization, not group realization. Future, more advanced Conference work will, I think, confirm this intuitive idea of groups of people simultaneously dreaming the same dream.

The exploration of the Tarot is very similar to dream work but has a distinct advantage: one can create an instantaneous dream merely by shuffling the cards and laying out the deck in a predetermined pattern.

The Tarot operates primarily through the symbolic, nonrational aspects of consciousness, the same state from which dreams communicate. The quality and accuracy of the Tarot interpretation depends solely upon the *querent*'s own ability, because it is only a reflection of the focus or level of consciousness of the inquirer. The Tarot is an excellent teacher, because as the user advances in expanded awareness it reflects this expansion. Therefore, the Tarot responds uniquely to each individual and never teaches more than the person is capable of receiving. One hears repeatedly about the Tarot that if a person were confined to a prison cell for life without parole, with only a Tarot deck, that person could gain the knowledge of the entirety of human experience, not only in the past but in the future as well!

No one knows the origin of the Tarot cards. Teachers of metaphysics often refer to the ancient Egyptians and the Hermetic School as the originators, but the earliest decks thus far discovered are European and from around the fourteenth century. Our modern playing cards are derived from the early Tarot decks, so at least fifty-two of the seventy-eight cards will be familiar to those who wish to explore this technique.

The Tarot consists of four suits, called the *minor arcana*, and each suit has fourteen cards — an ace through ten, a page, a knight, a queen and a king. The page through king are called court cards. The suits are divided into the wands (equivalent to clubs), the pentacles (diamonds), the swords (spades) and the cups (hearts). Thus there is a total of fifty-six cards in the minor arcana.

The *major arcana*, of twenty-one cards, bears the roman numerals I through XXI, representing life principles beyond the ordinary human levels. The final card in the Tarot deck, the Fool, is numbered zero, stands alone in neither arcana and is probably the most enigmatic of all. Some manufacturers supply, in addition, two blank cards to protect the top and bottom of the pack when not in use. Each of the seventy-eight cards displays a distinctive, individual picture.

I have selected the Rider Tarot deck, conceived by Arthur Edward Waite, for both Conference work and my own personal exploration for an essential reason: it offers the most literal representation of both outer and inner dream realities. There are many other decks, most of which have sprung up in recent years, but none of them touch the literal quality that I find so helpful in making the jump from the Tarot cards to what I call the Tarot of Life. The Egyptian, Witches, Aquarian and Mayan decks, although aesthetically beautiful, are designed with greater emphasis on geometric form or mystical symbols and are too abstract for my purposes.

As originally designed, each Tarot card represents a facet of the total life experience, from the mundane to the spiritual heights. Each card, like a dream, contains many symbols, which may be more or less obvious, depending upon the perspective of the viewer. Both the colors used and the numbering are important, because they are based on ancient principles derived from numerology and mystical teachings about colors. Every detail is significant in the interpretation of the card or cards; and in the process of interpretation, the outer mind sharpens its ability to see all the detail without losing the impression of the card as a whole.

As a channel to the understanding of human consciousness, in both its conscious and unconscious aspects, the Tarot has few peers. Even the *I Ching*, as magnificent a teacher as it is, cannot, in my opinion, make one aware of such psychological defenses as projection, nor tie in dream states, to the degree the Tarot can. In other areas they are on a par, that is, teaching both synchronicity — with insight into past, present and future — and the ancient wisdoms.

The Tarot (like the *I Ching*) is based on the assumption that the cards (or the coins or yarrow sticks used to divine the *I Ching* hexagram) are not separate from the consciousness of the inquirer. The querent's Beingness and the cards are in relationship to each other beyond the outer mind's ideas of time and space. The cards and the querent influence each other. The querent's higher awareness knows the final layout already — *before* the cards are shuffled. The higher dimensions of the querent's consciousness also know the answer to the question the querent is asking, and the shuffling and laying out of the cards is merely an act in linear time, a mechanism that establishes the channel to the higher levels of awareness. The same holds true for casting the coins or yarrow sticks in working with the *I Ching*. For readers who have difficulty accepting this concept, the parapsychological laboratories at Duke University and the University of California at Davis — and, for that matter, all parapsychological laboratories throughout the world — have voluminous evidence that certain people can consistently foretell almost exactly the sequence of a series of the twenty-five specially designed cards used in parapsychological work. Fewer can tell the exact or nearly exact sequence of cards one or two shuffles ahead, and a very rare person can predict the exact sequence of fifty-two cards of a regular playing-card deck in a future sequence, one or several shuffles ahead.

Whether one is calling the sequence of a deck that has been shuffled but not yet seen or whether one is predicting the sequence several shuffles ahead, the same mechanism of consciousness is involved. It is the ability to see or to have the future impressed upon one's awareness. To put it in other terms, our ordinary awareness is always in the past in relationship to expanded awareness. The higher levels simply utilize time and space as the outer organizational levels on which to display that which is not involved with time and space! The rare, talented individuals mentioned above do not need the Tarot or the *I Ching* as vehicles to expanded awareness. They have direct access, an attribute that greater numbers of humans will have developed in centuries to come.

We must realize that just as the physical body is not as it appears to be, time and space are not what the outer mind conceives them to be. All is energy interaction in a timeless state, and the apparent material plane is only a manifestation of one focus of the psyche. So, however incredible the theory of the Tarot may seem to the rational mind, the fact is that the rational mind is not a good judge of the question.

Somehow, that which creates us moment by moment also

creates the cards moment by moment, and in relationship to expanded awareness we and the cards are both in the past because all manifestations now are the results of processes and creations moments ago. Remember, in the dream reality every object, even though it appears to be separate and distinct from the observer, is a creation of some aspect of the dreamer's consciousness.

The Tarot is one of the best tools I know both for rapid insight into personal motives, time and space relationships and defenses that prevent the interpretation of the cards, and for reconditioning emotional responses, augmenting the intuitive faculty, restructuring personal belief systems and beginning access to more universal levels of awareness.

I have used the Tarot at the close of personal consultations, asking it to reveal to my outer mind any dynamics, overlooked in the session, that might be important. To my amazement, it often turns up a critical dynamic that has been totally unseen till then.

In the latter part of 1972, I was given my first Tarot deck. It had belonged to an elderly spiritual teacher who had died. His widow gave me the deck but suggested that I consult with it and ask its permission before using the cards. I was terribly excited, because I knew that I understood the Tarot at a deep level without having to train myself in its use. According to the mechanical techniques I really did know, I dutifully imbued the deck with my vibration, carefully shuffled the cards and held the question before my consciousness: "Do I have permission to use these cards?" When I laid the cards out in the traditional Celtic pattern, the layout clearly told me not to use the cards. Undaunted, I reshuffled the pack, really imbuing the cards with my vibration and again did a layout. Slightly more emphatically, the cards appeared to answer: "Not now." My rational mind refused to accept this answer, and, figuring that the odds were favorable for a positive response on the next layout, I again shuffled the deck and laid out the cards. This time some of the really negative cards began to show up, and the answer clearly was no!

What is a beginner querent into metaphysical realms to do but reshuffle the deck and try again? This time the answer came back, "NO! NO! NO!" Altogether I tried seven times, and each layout was more deprecating than the last one. I finally capitulated and, putting the cards away, did not touch a Tarot deck again until August 1976, when I was given another deck. My excitement was rekindled, but the memory of the previous encounter added a touch of anxiety. On the first layout, the response from this second deck was a strong affirmation, and my deeper exploration of the Tarot began.

I now realize that my work with all such tools and techniques—including palmistry, graphology, astrology, pendulum work — crystal ball work, tea leaf reading and radionics — had to be deferred until I had completed the development of a direct channel into these states of awareness through the process of meditation and the Inner Teacher, both topics to be covered in a later chapter. There is a very real danger of displacing the power of direct consciousness awareness on to any of these objects or vehicles, in which case they can actually interfere with the opening of the direct channel.

Initially, dreams, the Tarot and the *I Ching* are to make one more self-aware. As with any good teacher, they fall away as one enters more deeply into the states of direct knowledge.

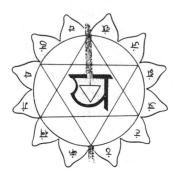

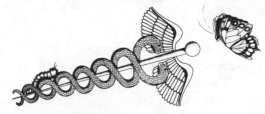

CHAPTER FIVE

Lona Brugh Joy
and Eunice Jean Hurt

*A Radiance of Love
heightens beyond one's ability to conceive.*

To be quickened by Love, the unconditional radiance that emanates from the heart chakra, moves even the most skeptical person into the Transformational Process. It is the energy that uplifts downcast eyes, heals the pain of years of struggle, nourishes the soul in its venture to unite with the spirit, inspirits the mundane and transmutes that which is not to be into that which is to be. It is the essence of the cohesive force that binds all things to God. This Love is nonemotional, nonsexual and nonmental. It has the power to spiritualize instantaneously, imbuing each individual with an expanded experience of universal relationship and universal values. The sensation is one of Divinity, and it does not matter whether rational states comprehend. This Love is the energy that sweeps one toward home, a return to the embrace with God.

    The awakening of Love in the physical body is sheer ecstasy, a palpable bliss that is incomprehensible to the everyday mind. Suddenly the concepts of spiritual awakening, the Divine, the world vision and the Aquarian Age are experienced directly. The deepest yearning a soul can sense is satisfied, the fear of commitment erased without trace: one's total Beingness is released into the first taste of a Unity that transcends those ideas about the integration of mind, body and spirit that are so lavishly discussed but so rarely experienced.

One's purposing emerges clearly in consciousness; the windmills of the mind cease as the true beauty of humanity in its coherent form becomes a whole and is seen as a whole. This Love is sensed as intrinsic and fundamental, and, once ignited, it requires no external source for its propagation. Every religion of the world has at its center this awakening experience, the reconnection to the Whole. Sexual, emotional and mental love all require externals for continuation, but not Love, not the fourth level of awareness where Love stands alone, totally inclusive, unconditioned and unconditional.

The experience, in sequence, of two remarkable external teachers, my mother and Eunice, was what fully precipitated this awareness in me.

My mother, Lona Brugh Joy, was a rainbow of delicate white skin, light blue eyes, auburn hair, long red-painted fingernails, brown mascaraed eyelashes, light brown eyebrows artistically curved and etched. She enjoyed garments of spring colors, and wall colorings of light gold and ivory with splashes of oranges, pinks and greens for accent. She was like a china doll and small in stature — five feet — but ever so big in determination and strength when provoked or prodded. She raised three sons with balances of force and love so delicate as to surpass my ability to describe it. Above all, she was consistent and unpreferential, showering the gifts of her Beingness equally on all three sons; and the ground rules were clear.

Mother was in charge — until the inevitable late-teenage rebellion of male offspring supervened. It was a difficult transition for her, because she knew that no woman would possibly be able to nourish her sons in the manner she had so unselfishly maintained throughout the years of our rearing. Even later when she fully accepted our wives, she never lost an opportunity to teach them how to work with and to understand each of us.

When Mother was angry, she was angry, and no one escaped knowing or feeling it. She did not become upset often but when she did, silence and withdrawal were the only ways to respond to her. There was a stubborn streak in her that was awesome to behold, beautiful to see when she was fighting to get us through illness or educational obstacles but not so pleasant to us when we were heading in directions not to her liking. She saw our highest potentials as what she was there to aid, encourage and augment; and she never confused our highest potentials with her own personal dreams. We were not extensions of her unfulfilled desires but rather the natural fulfillment of her life. Just the family together was enough, no one else was needed to share in the humor, deep conversation, love, conflict, entertainment and a sense of belonging. Of all of these, humor and love played the greatest roles. We could laugh and laugh over some of the most ridiculous things, even over the times when she would have us go over to the park to pick a willow switch that she would use on us when we had misbehaved.

She was a smart woman. The long walk to and from the park, and the task of having to pick just the right switch, which would sting but not cut the skin, were more effective in punishment and in our understanding of why we were being punished than any talk or argument. There was ample time for us to think about what we had done. We never felt that she rejected us or our love, because when the switching was over we always understood why she had switched us and embraced her for it — maybe not right after the switching, but within a short period of time.

This first teacher of mine nourished all the sensitive and aesthetic values within me. Harmony in music, the arts and deeper spiritual values were developed under her guidance, although in the case of the spiritual values, her guidance was certainly not conventional. The mystery school teachings, rather than any of the encrusted orthodox approaches to religion, were, as she said, her cup of tea. She sought and always found the harmonious, whether in the latest theories in physics dealing with the atomic and subatomic particles or in trance mediums' reports of life after death.

Mother respected life forms in a way I am only now appreciating. She never killed flies, spiders or any small creature entering our home but carefully enmeshed them in towels and carried them outside. She admitted sometimes that, when she watered flowers and plants, she talked to them. When she cut flowers for inside the home, she "worked" silently with the plant so that it would release its flowering without pain. She understood what was natural and beautiful and surrounded herself with objects reflecting these qualities, whether in art form, written form or in physical-material form. In her later years, she would consciously place a thought of beauty in the place of that which was negative or, in her words, "not right."

She taught me that time was a belief system and not of universal importance. Something in the past could be corrected just as well as something in the present — and just as easily, too. The future was to be harmoniously created. She was not an intense intellectual thinker but instead used the intellectual insights of others to spark her intuitive creative imagination. To her, life was a school of experiences, and her most important task was to establish her children in fulfilling paths of endeavor.

She taught that illness was a misperception of an already perfect manifestation; it is the essential concept in mental healing. Her mental treatment of a problem went something like this: this (the problem) isn't, and this (her idea of perfection) is, and that's that. One would have to sense her energy field to understand why this form of thinking was all that her consciousness needed. She respected science and medicine but always worked from the metaphysical aspect because she felt that science and medicine were a bit behind the times. "Someday you will see the blending of science and medicine with the metaphysical," she said to me when I was a child. She lived long enough to enjoy the first fruits of this statement.

She was profoundly influenced by Ernest Holmes, Joseph

Murphy, Neville, Yogananda, the White books (Stuart Edward White), Swedenborg, Plato, Thomas Merton, Taylor Caldwell and the words of Jesus. She taught me how to enter a library and just let a book "pop out" into my awareness from the shelves; such a book always contained the most amazing information, often on a subject that I might have been working on for months without insight. She didn't believe in the concept of evil, other than recognizing it as a creation of confused areas of the human psyche. In her mind, Love and God were synonymous. God had no specific form, nor did Love. Each was infinite, inextricably fused and perdurable.

Mother ignited my interest in the metaphysical realms of thought, and we had long discussions late into the night on such matters. We never grew tired of this exploration. We shared with each other our creative insights, visions and conflicts. In my early adult life, it was a coexploration, much to our mutual satisfaction. Little escaped our attention and perusal. Looking back at this phase of my life, I most appreciate the overall experience of the training in both historical and present-day developments in the human quest toward unification with God and, most important, the training in the verbalizing of these matters.

Mother met Eunice at my wedding to Wendey in September 1972. At that ceremony she also turned over the reins of my spiritual development — not to my wife, but to Eunice, the minister who performed the ceremony. Eunice was inspiring, reassuring my first teacher (Mother) that this second teacher (Eunice) was her worthy successor, even though Eunice was dying of cancer and at that point had only two months to live.

In the late 1960s, when I was twenty-seven and studying internal medicine at the Mayo Clinic in Rochester, Minnesota, I had an intuitive flash that I would meet and study with a woman spiritual teacher in Los Angeles, California, at some time in my early thirties. In my earlier years, flashes of the future had been common — always prophetic, signaling major changes, usually years in advance. Even before I entered college to commence the prerequisites for medical school, one of these flashes had implied clearly that I wouldn't be practicing medicine after the age of thirty-five. The flash didn't indicate what I *would* be doing, but that part of the essential change that was to occur was present in my awareness even then, before I was twenty.

When I was twenty-nine, stationed at Balboa Naval Hospital in San Diego, California, the image of Eunice as the individual who was to be my teacher entered my awareness. The image of study in Los Angeles was confusing to me, because when I left Los Angeles at twenty-five to commence my internship at Johns Hopkins Hospital, I had vowed never to return.

Having grown up in Southern California, primarily in the Los Angeles area, I had found that life in a large, sprawling, smoggy, congested city could be uninspiring and, at times, downright depressing. On clear days my mood and judgments would change to embrace the beauty of the beaches, mountains, palm trees...and the delightful melting pot of cultures. There was also the craziness my drinking friends and I entered into on every night when exam time didn't demand a more disciplined attitude toward studies. That period in my life was like a whirlpool for me. To my amazement I was able to graduate with honors from medical school and at the same time graduate from the mad Los Angeles nightlife of the early sixties. It was tinsel and loud music, fluorescent lights and wildly uninhibited people, and I was not naive about life in my early twenties.

But something deeper was beginning to emerge, because I found absolutely no fulfillment in such a frenetic existence. In my internship at Johns Hopkins, I was too busy to know that Baltimore even existed, but later, as a resident in internal medicine, with more time to relax, I found the same pattern there that I had uncovered in Los Angeles. Obviously, the pattern was internal not external.

Later, my two years at the Mayo Clinic were probably the most serene of my life, because in Rochester, Minnesota, there is absolutely nothing to do at night but study. I centered my entire attention on medicine. I matured into a physician while I was there, and I would have stayed on to practice medicine at the clinic had it not been for my military obligation, which took me to San Diego, foreshadowing the pull back to Los Angeles. During my last year of naval service, I received an offer to enter into partnership with two outstanding and highly respected internists in, of all places, downtown Los Angeles. My admiration and respect for these two physicians outweighed my feelings against the city, and I therefore returned.

Before I describe my first meeting with Eunice, some relevant preliminaries are needed. I had had numerous experiences with the paranormal before medical school, but that entire aspect of my being ceased abruptly the moment I entered medical school and started the formal training to become a physician.

Earlier, as an undergraduate, I had often been able to intuit an examination the evening before; and sometimes I simply allowed the answers to test questions to flow into my awareness during the examination, even on subjects I hadn't studied. As a medical student, however, I received no such paranormal aid, and I had to develop the mental faculties of memorization and logical deduction. It was as if a brick wall had suddenly been built between my intuitive areas and the outer rational areas of the thought process. Only later did I realize that that brick wall was precisely what I needed at that time. Without my psi abilities, I had to study at more intense levels to learn orthodox medicine, and I learned it well. Most important, the experience gave me a thorough grounding in rational deductive thought processes.

Actually, I didn't find the study of medicine overwhelmingly difficult; it was exciting, intensely interesting and moving. I was awed by the human body and even more awed by the problems that befall it. Human suffering was a deep mystery that piqued my intellectual curiosity. I was often moved to tears when suffering was assuaged, whether through treatment or through death. I particularly loved delivering infants into the world, and I dreaded the encounter with the dying and their families. Acute diseases rallied my entire armamentarium, while chronic diseases frustrated and depleted my energies. In the initial phases of my professional life, death and the incurable were emotionally unacceptable to me because they indicated failure on my part. I still battle the "incurable" and ideas about death — but not alone; I have invited the patient to do battle along with me.

The wall between the intuitive and the rational had begun to weaken during my residency at the Mayo Clinic. When I finished my residency, the wall crumbled. My interest in metaphysics was rekindled as a deep yearning to explore higher states of consciousness. The awareness that I was to meet Eunice quickened me during my first year and a half in private practice.

In October 1971, a male patient who came in for a routine checkup suggested that I might enjoy meeting his spiritual teacher. We had already talked briefly about metaphysical healing concepts, but I wasn't yet prepared to accept his invitation. After all, there are so many funny cults in Southern California. (One cartoon puts it beautifully with a signpost on a desert highway: "You are now leaving California — resume normal behavior.") But when my patient mentioned that the teacher was a "she," and that her name was Eunice Hurt, I was overwhelmed with excitement. *My God*, I thought, *the intuitive flash was correct*. But I didn't drop my stethoscope and dash over to meet her. I knew that I was going to study with her, and I knew the timing of our meeting had nothing to do with my personal need or excitement. In fact, I wasn't to meet her for six weeks.

The moment came on a Saturday afternoon in December 1971, when the patient called and said that Eunice would like to meet me. I was nervous, because my outer thinking was that she might not accept me. The pull toward this woman was not normal; it was paranormal, and I knew it.

She was living in a small house in Van Nuys, a suburban community in the San Fernando Valley, the "bedroom" of Los Angeles. When I entered the living room, where she was seated, my heart pounded and my palms were perspiring. She stood, looked me over carefully, then laughed and opened her arms to me. The radiance of her Beingness was Love made manifest. I was swept into a state of ecstasy. It was an internal ecstasy, because I was almost motionless, caught in a state of sensing the Divine, while my outer mind was left contending with appearances.

Eunice was forty-six years old, but what I was feeling was an ageless "old" soul, a temple of ancient wisdoms with a presence I did not have to try to feel but that enfolded and uplifted my own. We didn't speak for several minutes. Then, with perfect eye contact, a mutual "yes" was whispered.

I cried when I returned home. In fact, I cried all that night and all the next day. The tears were not of sadness nor of grief nor of pain nor of suffering; they were the tears of inexplicable joy. I had recognized her Beingness, and when I use the word *recognize*, I mean the deep recognition that is so very rarely experienced — the remeeting with a soul one has loved and respected in past lifetimes. She was brother, teacher, mother, sister, father, son and wife. She was spiritual coworker, fellow Buddhist disciple, Zen master and ancient Egyptian teacher of the healing arts. Our souls were entwined over many lifetimes, always for the purpose of helping to awaken one or the other, and usually to help one or the other to cross over when death came. A week before she died, nine months after I started to study with her, she told me this last detail — a detail I already knew. She will be present at my own death.

Meeting somebody from a past lifetime is actually a very common occurrence, but one that is filtered from the outer mind, which has absolutely no memory of prior existences. But our unconscious does not deny nor can it possibly deny, that which is fundamental to the essence of Life. I do not intend to dwell on concepts of reincarnation nor to develop convincing proofs. When one reaches a certain level of development, this knowledge enters the awareness and needs no rationalization.

In December 1971 and January 1972, I attended the last four weekly evening sessions of a series of sixteen classes Eunice was giving to the public. They were followed by eight more classes, closed sessions, with attendance by her invitation only. Much of the content dealt with group-healing concepts, dream interpretation, metaphysical principles and the teachings of Jesus. The deepest level of teaching did not begin until March 1972 when, according to an impress she had received, she took a few of her students into experiential realms of awareness I had only read about.

By the time she finished with me, I had thrown down every last remnant of skepticism. I was defenseless, because her mastery of psi phenomena was nothing short of miraculous. Her gifts of telepathy, clairvoyance and precognition were accurate and proved. She could, if she desired, generate a force field that could knock over a huge and powerful man. Neither her students' thoughts nor their actions were unavailable to her. There could be no games or deception, because she knew the truth of one's Beingness. As she told each one of us at the outset, it was no trivial task to take on the responsibility of training even one student, let alone twelve. Because of our mutual commitment, her awareness of each one of us was acute twenty-four hours a day.

I had never experienced Unconditional Love until the moment I met Eunice. There were no strings attached, and no judgments issued from her being about any of the more unsavory aspects of her students. She saw what she called the Divinity of each soul: the personality level and the confusion of the outer mind were unnecessary to the induction process. She was the great awakener, and she knew it. The last three years of her life were ones of ministry and teaching. Even her children became secondary to this task.

Born and raised on a farm in the Midwest, Eunice in her earlier years had experienced the poverty of the Depression era. She related many episodes of the paranormal, including actual physical body levitation, before adolescence. I am unaware of most of the details of her outer life — working her way through school, five marriages that ended in divorce, her outer training in metaphysics and the various places she had worked as a secretary in Los Angeles. Her public lecture work and private counseling sessions had begun approximately two years before we met.

She had an excellent mind and was quite capable of conversing in the areas of advanced mathematics, physics, history and philosophy. Although deeply knowledgeable in both the Old and the New Testaments, she was eclectic in her approach to religious principles. She drew from the Buddhist sutras, Sufi concepts, Hindu teachings, the Cabala, Hermetic philosophy, Zen Buddhist koans and Islamic teachings; but fundamentally she always used a Christian model on which to display these other teachings and principles. Even though she was profoundly religious, there was always the balance of her sharp intellect, which could cut to pieces a skeptic whose doubts were based on intellectual grounds.

To the external eye, she was a hard-working secretary raising a teenage son and daughter. She smoked two packs of cigarettes a day; used little, if any, alcohol; loved all kinds of food; occasionally fasted; had traveled little outside the United States; loved a good joke; could swear appropriately; dressed conventionally; bleached her hair; was very frightened of water, from ocean to swimming pool; tended to be mildly overweight; enjoyed conversation for hours on end; was a very strong fighter for what she believed in; cared little for animals and plants; could play like a child; did not personally like everyone she met; and could lose her temper, particularly with her children. That was Eunice at her personality level.

But when she blended with more expanded portions of her Beingness, as she could do in a blink of an eye, she was saintlike, a totally different entity, whose words were like liquid light and whose presence was sheer manna.

In metaphysical terms, she had developed the ability to blend with her high self instantaneously, demonstrating Christ consciousness—the essence of Love.

Thus, Eunice was a real person, with problems just like those of any other human being, but with one exception: she was awake. There was no need in her to meet the expectations others may have desired her to meet, to deceive people by displaying only her sainted pattern or to gain personal power over others with the use of her gifts.

When she was in her ordinary awareness, she was a delight. When she was channeling spiritual principles and energies from another dimension, she was mind-boggling. It was through the difference between Eunice's ordinary awareness and her more expanded Beingness that I later learned to see that the personality level is like a garment. It can serve the purpose of developing experiences, but when it is no longer useful, when it can take one no further, it is to be discarded as a garment is discarded, as the body is discarded when it is time to enter another plane. Once I had learned experientially that I did not have to stay in the personality level, once I knew that there were alternatives, I could begin the resolution of problems configurated at the personality level.

The intensity of her teaching, so unselfishly showered on the small groups of individuals during the last nine months of her life, cannot be summarized fully — or even shared partially — without distortion. I can say that it was like riding on the back of a winged horse as she took each of us into dimension after dimension of consciousness beyond the ordinary, through the power of her inducting field, sharing wisdoms in the art of healing and in the achievement of self-realization.

Meditation was basic to her teachings. Anyone who could not meditate missed the "inner-plane" experience. In my case, meditation freed my identity from my outer mind. The impossible became possible, and the insoluble became its own solution.

Keep in mind that during my study with Eunice I was a totally orthodox internist, practicing the subspecialities of pulmonary and cardiac medicine in addition to general internal medicine. I had not come into the awareness of body energy fields, chakras and the transmutation of diseased tissue. Traditional medical concepts dominated my thinking as they dominated my practice of medicine. I not only was on the teaching faculty of the Hospital of the Good Samaritan Medical Center, but was also an assistant clinical professor of medicine at the Los Angeles County/University of Southern California Medical Center (L.A.County Hospital), teaching general and pulmonary medicine to medical students, interns and residents.

In July 1972, Eunice coughed up some blood. A mass

lesion was noted in the left hilar region of her lungs. Within three days surgery was performed, but the prognosis was poor. The lesion was highly malignant, but not, as one might have suspected, the type of cancer associated with her smoking. It was a scar cancer, developing out of scar tissue associated with an old granulomatous disease, probably a fungal infection.

The dichotomy of Eunice's Beingness became evident. The personality level was angered, frustrated that her life was going to end just as she was reaching the prime of her teachings. Her concern for her children dominated her thinking as she reluctantly began to put her affairs into order. Her outer mind, feeling trapped in an uncontrollable circumstance, cried out in anguish. The fear of pain occasionally obsessed her and made her plead with me to reassure her that I would not withhold narcotics.

She recuperated from the lung surgery in the guest cottage in which she had trained our group in spiritual work. There she related a supervivid dream in which a station wagon, in which she was driving us all to an unknown destination, broke down after climbing a steep hill. After the vehicle coasted down the hill into an old gasoline station, a mechanic inspected the engine and told her there was nothing to do, that it was irreparably damaged. In the dream she announced to us that we were all going to have to get out of the car and walk the rest of the way.

When she finished relating the dream there was silence in the room. Whether the others were able to allow the interpretation of this dream into their awareness, I do not know; but I saw its significance and discussed it with Eunice in a private session after that class. She was going to die. Her body was beyond cure, and all of us were going to have to find our own paths without her help. The dream occurred in spite of the evidence that after her surgery the cancerous process was not detectable. In her heightened awareness, she told me that she had deliberately related the dream to prepare her students for her death, which would take place toward the end of the year.

She also told me that earlier in the year she had had an impress that she was going to be called to a distant land, a foreign country. Her outer mind had interpreted this to mean a trip to the Far East. Now she knew that termination of her physical form was to take place. She realized that her commitment in this lifetime had been fulfilled: she had been here to awaken certain individuals, and she had done so. She had no fear of the death process and, in fact, would instruct me in the preparation for her death at the appropriate time. Meanwhile, she refused chemotherapy and radiation, because, though her outer mind clung to the hope of a cure, she rejected palliation and demanded either complete cure or death.

There was still no postoperative evidence of the cancerous process when she married Wendey and me on September 30, 1972. Wendey and I flew to Tobago for our honeymoon and returned to the United States three weeks later to attend a medical convention in Denver, Colorado. One of her students telephoned me there to say that Eunice had been taken to the hospital with abdominal pain. Wendey and I immediately flew back to Los Angeles.

When I examined Eunice, I found the cancer everywhere — in her abdomen, her neck and in her groins. One of her physicians had told her that it was of no concern and Eunice, in almost a childlike state of consciousness, believed him. I looked at her with tears in my eyes, but she wanted to know the truth, so I told her: she had less than a month to live. She thanked me, because it made it clear that the preparation for her crossing had to begin.

Because the pain was so excruciating, she asked me to begin the process of using morphine to place her in coma so that her death would be accelerated by pneumonia, something I had on occasion done for others who were nearing death. I promised her I would do just that and ordered morphine injections to be given every four hours around the clock, even if she seemed to be comfortable, asleep or otherwise not in pain. It didn't work. Despite very large doses, she would not enter a coma; and finally, after three days, I spoke to her about her lack of cooperation. She laughed and said there must be more work to do. Even if her outer mind wanted to escape the nightmare of pain, her soul was not ready to leave.

Then she accomplished one of her miraculous displays. In twenty-four hours, she made the masses in her neck subside completely. She stated emphatically that she did not wish to die in a hospital, that she wanted to go home. She also wanted to demonstrate that the healing of her body was possible, and that in dying she was going to yield to an inner calling.

We took her back to the guest cottage, hired a special nurse to be with her and awaited the inevitable. Eunice went on teaching, counseling each of us until the last week.

On a late November morning Eunice died, but not before telling her nurse that she saw two angels standing on either side of a man with a Christ-like appearance who was beckoning to her. She raised from the bed, sitting up with her arms outstretched, then rested back on the pillow and died.

Yes, Eunice had instructed me in the art of dying, but my attachment to her on the personality level had prevented me from fully appreciating at the time what a rich and valuable experience it was. With her death came physical grief and only then the full implication of her teaching. She had given each one of us the "keys to the Kingdom." We could continue to search for another teacher, but her teachings were amazingly complete. Another person might phrase the principles differently, but the essentials were one and the same. We had to get out of the car and walk.

I began that walk by setting aside at least an hour each morning to enter into a deep meditative state of consciousness. Sometimes it would mean getting up at four in the morning, after completing long days at the hospital and in the office and retiring at midnight. I knew the path was internal and not external. There could and would be no further external teacher. I had been given the gift of a lifetime, and I knew it. The manifestation of my own self-awareness was my responsibilty and no one else's.

How many times have I observed people sitting in living rooms, lecture halls or in mountain retreats, listening to an inspired teacher. Some of these people had been doing the same thing for a year, five years, even forty years. After all that time they still persist in failing to realize that the critical step is in being, not in what is spoken about being. Action must be taken, and that action is inside.

Almost two months to the day after Eunice's death, I found my Inner Teacher—a state of consciousness that continues to teach me today. It is not a manifestation of Eunice or of anybody else that I recognize in my outer mind. Its presence is radiant; and its wisdom, inspiring.

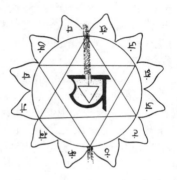

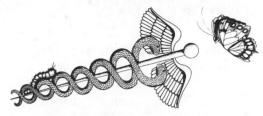

CHAPTER SIX

Six Quantum Leaps

Nothing is as it appears
to be, even when one is certain.

In my Transformational Process there have been six "quantum leaps"—experiential insights that have radically and suddenly altered my perception of reality. As I use the expression here, a "quantum leap" is a jump from one level of realization to another without passing through an intervening development to arrive at the new awareness. Up to a certain point in time, you hold one set of beliefs; and in the next instant, you experience a whole new perspective. In any such case, you cannot comprehend the validity of the new experience unless you relinquish an idea, or many ideas, that you have held till then.

In my case it took over thirty years to establish the foundation on which these leaps in awareness could take place. All of them were slow in brewing, were accelerated by the process of meditation and were infused with a sense of expansion and deeper truth about the manifest plane and its relationship to the psyche and to the spirit.

For me the six major insights were:
1. The relativity of all reality and the importance of state-bound consciousness
2. The differentiation of sequential experiences from simultaneous experiences and the real meaning of the now moment
3. The breakdown of the skin-bound consciousness
4. The realization of the difference between thought forms and essences
5. The resolution of the death space
6. The experience of Unconditional Love

This chapter is a distillation of the innumerable experiences and contemplations that brought about these insights.

RELATIVE REALITY

Albert Einstein had the genius to take the obvious and validate it with mathematics. Without him, people might have gone on forever denying in their intellects what they had known for eons in their lives: two individuals observing the same event from two different points in space do not experience the same reality. Going even further than Einstein, I would state that two people who observed the same event from the same point in space at the same point in time (if it were physically possible) would not experience the same reality. Why? Because each person's focus of awareness is different, so that no two people can possibly draw the same conclusions. Each individual's consciousness is unique, not only in its historical background, but also in the kind and degree of its filtration. Experiences of the manifest plane are always, and can only be, relative to the perspective of the viewer. There are, therefore, as many different realities occurring simultaneously as there are foci of awareness. In regard to any event, there are as many realities as there are observers, and each reality is equally valid.

I usually illustrate this point by inscribing in space the largest circle it is possible to draw with my finger. That circle could conceivably include the entire universe, but for the moment let's limit it to a circle with a radius as long as my arm. Now, put a dot—the tiniest of dots—anywhere in that circle. We let the space within the circle symbolically represent your total possible awareness, while the little dot represents your awareness in any given moment. Now, using the same radius, transform that circle into a sphere and the dot into a tiny sphere. We now have a model in three-dimensional reality.

Now imagine, inside this larger sphere, many small spheres, the size of marbles, representing each and every possible state of awareness. The tiny dot-sphere representing your momentary outer awareness can go into any one of these marble-sized spheres. The first such sphere you enter might be labeled "conditioned ideas about reality." While you are in this space, everything fits in with that label, and nothing contradicts it. You next enter a sphere labeled "neurotic state," with the subtitle "fear of rejection." All reality you perceive from this focus of awareness confirms this perspective—you are an object to be rejected—and nothing denies it. Then, let's say your tiny sphere of awareness enters a marble-sized sphere called "depression." No matter what you perceive there, everything feels and looks bleak and dark, and despair and pain get worse and worse. And so on, through as many labels as you can imagine. The ordinary human awareness goes through just such a process—but in a more complex way, because memory is a dimension always superimposed on the moment's experience so that the experience of the present moment is altered even further.

The process of enlightenment is the process of acquiring the ability to expand that tiny sphere of awareness to include more and more of the marble-sized spheres and thereby to include a larger and larger portion of the large sphere. When you reach the point where your awareness at any given moment includes the entire larger sphere, you have achieved illumination.

Many individuals have entered a space labeled "expanded awareness" and called the experience "enlightenment." But, because their individual focus was not expanded, they have not been truly enlightened. They have, it is true, had a peak experience in spaces not easily penetrated by the aware focus; but their real task, still before them, is to expand their awareness to encompass that peak-experience space, and all the others, *all in the same moment*. A peak experience is far from enlightenment.

The more inclusive an individual's aware consciousness, the greater his or her soul development.

I also illustrate relative reality with the idea of a series of slides. First is the perspective of the earth as viewed from the ground. One could get lost just trying to grasp the myriad details of Los Angeles—even spend a lifetime or two studying its aspects. To make the project more difficult, it is constantly changing—with new roads and buildings added and old ones removed, and so on. One's entire focus of awareness could be spent in this activity and not even get into neighboring Southern California areas, or to San Francisco, New Delhi, or Paris. This situation is analogous to being stuck in a psychological set or a fixation of awareness: while you are in it, nothing is going to make you believe that there is any other possibility of experience. Your focus on a problem or situation is so close that you cannot see anything outside it. In fact, our laws of relativity would state that the closer you are to any object, whether material or psychological, the larger or more vast it will be — not seem, but be! In fact, if your focus of awareness were to penetrate a single atom, that atom would take on the appearance and the dimensions of an entire solar system. (Your problems get bigger when you focus on them.)

The next few slides would show the earth from an orbiting satellite. Not only can you now see a far vaster portion of the whole, but the appearance of the ground is radically altered. Roadways in and out of cities can be seen. The relationship of one city to another can easily be grasped. Mountains, rivers, oceans, lakes, cities, roads and other topographical features now appear in relationship to one another. Egypt from the air and Egypt from the ground are two different experiences. The former is a ribbon of green meandering through a vast desert, while the latter is a mass of teeming towns and village-farms extending out on either side of a large muddy river.

The next slides would show the earth as seen from 100,000 miles away, progressively farther and farther, and eventually show the earth from the moon. From there it is staggering to conceive of the entire history of humankind, up to and including this very moment's developments, as taking place on that small multicolored globe. Billions of people are swarming over the planet, and not one can be seen from this perspective. (And where are your problems now?)

We next view slides of the moon as seen from its surface, then go on to Mercury, Venus, Mars, Jupiter, Saturn, Uranus, Neptune and Pluto; and finally we move out into the galaxy and beyond. From this perspective, all that remains of the earth and the totality of human endeavor isn't even perceptible to the eye, but infinite other perceptions and experiences in awareness are—including the possibility of focusing on another sun, with its planets and their life forms, perhaps more advanced than ours.

There are billions of suns just in our own galaxy. More than one hundred million of them are thought to have planetary solar systems similar to ours. Since there are billions of galaxies, the probability of life in the known universe is high.

While light from our own star, the sun, reaches us in about 8.3 minutes, light from the nearest star outside our solar system takes 4.3 years. The farther we are away from these distant objects in the known universe, the farther back in time are the events that we perceive—up to perhaps ten billion years for stars at the farthest observable reaches of space.

As long as we can perceive and conceive only in linear models, it will be more than four years before we can know that anything major has happened at the nearest star in our own galaxy. Fortunately, there are alternatives to linear models, as I will demonstrate in the sections on simultaneity. Most important, however, is that a change of perspective in thought changes actual time and actual physical relationships. This suggestion may be a clue as to how a change in attitude about a disease process can influence the course of that disease process. From all that has been said, we may even infer that the disease process may be affected not only by changes of attitude in the patient, but also by changes in the attitude of the physician, healer, therapist or anyone else who is a part of the patient's consciousness.

We are beings of an undetermined number of dimensions exploring the third and fourth dimensions. These three or four dimensions are a school for gods in which we learn in slow motion the consequences of thought. This conception of us and our world is diametrically opposed to the more common idea that we are third- and fourth-dimensional beings who are trying in vain to comprehend the n dimensions of reality.

Another example of relative reality, which we have already considered, is the interpretation of the Tarot cards. Here again, the perspective determines or creates what one sees. In a group of twenty or so people, I usually demonstrate this phenomenon by having one individual name the card he or she most dislikes. The other participants then find the same card in their own decks and study it for a few minutes. After the person who selected the card gives his or her interpretation of it, I ask the group, "How many of you saw the card change as the interpretation was given?" Up go the hands. Most of the people always see their own initial perspective of the card — and therefore their experience of it — change into something similar to what the first person reported seeing. To emphasize this relativity, I ask each person to relate what he or she first saw in the card, and with each sharing, the card seems to change magically for all of them. This experience is only the beginning of understanding how perspective determines what one experiences. And twenty people encounter only the bare possibilities contained in just one card.

In teaching psychotherapeutic work, I extend this relativity concept to show the importance of seeing another's perspective — that is, the way the individual is configurating the problem or problems. This perspective is then put into relationship to the therapist's various perspectives, which hold the potential resolution. When the problems are projected onto the Tarot cards, the client has the opportunity to observe how differently the card appears when the therapist presents alternative views. In my psychotherapeutic work I do not just give options to the clients. My fundamental purpose is to enable the clients to learn to see options for themselves.

Two personal examples demonstrate how my own attitudinal shifts changed my perception of events.

In the first seventeen-day Conference at Sky Hi Ranch, which I presented in September 1975, I played for the group an English translation of the record of the *Bhagavad-Gita*, a twenty-five-hundred-year-old Hindu epic poem from India. On hearing it, I was enraptured, truly ecstatic, and so I played the identical record again in the Conference of January 1976. This time I was enraged by what I heard. I was angry over almost every statement in it. Then, during one of those moments of anger, I suddenly realized what was going on. I brought the September experience back to my mind. How could I, in a past moment, have experienced this record as one of the most beautiful and, in this moment, barely tolerate it? Then it dawned on me: since the poem was innocent and the record the same, something must have happened inside me to produce the second, diametrically opposite response. When I shifted my focus of awareness to a heightened state, I again experienced the harmony of the poem.

When the record was over, most of the members of the group said that they detested it and were angered by it. In them its religious associations had stirred up deep-seated resentment. I experienced a sudden insight into the power of group consciousness: even though all the participants had been lying quietly on the floor, listening to the record, I had been somehow swept up in their unspoken emotional responses. As some participants with powerful energy fields reacted in anger, the rest of the group was inducted into the same emotional perspective, and I was caught by it, too — until I realized what was happening and, enabled by my training, blocked the induction.

The group's mood was depressed, resentful and angry. I then asked the participants to form a circle and shift their awareness to Unconditional Love. Two minutes after they did so, the energy of the group — and all the energy in the room — was transmuted into harmony. It was a profound experience, especially for me, because I knew from experience that people usually take hours or days to work through feelings of anger and resentment. Now, having listened to the *Bhagavad-Gita* at least six times, I have responded in so many different ways that I wonder whether I shall ever hear what it is actually saying — and whether what it is saying is even the point.

The second example to demonstrate the consequences of an attitudinal shift concerns my feelings about my facial asymmetry. One of my ears is noticeably lower than the other, and so is one of my eyes. I became aware of this imbalance at about the age of ten; and to make it less obvious, I had learned to tilt my head a certain way and to comb my hair to minimize the apparent disproportion. Still it was almost intolerable to my ego that this disharmony existed. Then several years ago I came across an article that pointed out that mystics often have distortions of the face, and when I then looked into the mirror I said, "It's not distorted enough!" My ego needs had completely shifted my perspective to a new behavior and feeling.

The phenomenon of state-bound consciousness is closely connected to relative reality. As you already know, ordinary consciousness is only one of many possibilities. It is primarily a trained state of mind, a conditioned state. We have been told how and what to think and, for the most part, how to act. Ordinary consciousness is the one that perceives Los Angeles as a city, whereas, when you see it from another state of consciousness, you can't see where it begins or ends or, therefore, whether it exists. As a matter of fact, it *doesn't* exist — really. It exists only at a certain level of consciousness. No forms of life but the human have any idea that Los Angeles exists. Your ordinary awareness has vast experience and vast information available to it about this conditioned level, albeit this information may be compartmentalized within the normal or conventional states of consciousness.

The term "state-bound consciousness" means that the information known to one perspective or state of awareness is bound to that particular perspective or state of awareness and is generally unavailable to other perspectives or states.

When we dream at night, our consciousness is obviously in a different state from its ordinary waking state. Sometimes we can bring some of the dream experience back into the outer state of awareness but, for the most part, dream experiences are bound to the dream state and are unavailable to the outer mind. As a byproduct of meditation, however, one can develop the ability to shift from one state to another, and thus recapture dream experiences in all their detail. This phenomenon is one of the several reasons why I consider meditation to be empowering. It enables the mind to go into any state of consciousness and retrieve information that ordinarily can be experienced only at that level. Charles Tart of the University of California at Davis has devoted much of his energies to teaching and writing about the binding of information to the level in which it is first experienced.

In one experiment (not by Tart), medical students drank alcohol until they were drunk, and then they were trained. When they sobered up, they were tested on what they had learned while they were drunk. They did poorly but when the experimenters got them drunk again — and tested them *while* they were drunk — the students performed much better on the same material. Much of the information was entirely unavailable to them when they were sober.

Something similar occurs when individuals enter high states of consciousness through meditation or when the gift of channeling is achieved and the wisdom of the information received transcends ordinary awareness. When individuals return to ordinary awareness, most of the information is lost to the outer mind. Such is the case with many inspired teachers. When they are "in stream" — a term that denotes a shift to a more expanded awareness — they verbalize or channel information from that state of experience. If the stream of consciousness is broken — as by questions from students or by some other action — the connection is disrupted, the teacher's focus of consciousness shifts and the experiences of another level are lost, at least momentarily. The teacher may not even be able to tell the student what he or she was discussing. A tape recording, however, can sometimes recapture what was experienced in the higher state, and a master teacher can return at will to the state where the information is bound and rechannel it.

Inspired writers demonstrate the same phenomenon. When they reread their creative writing several days later, they often find that what they wrote seems to be not of themselves, as if it would be impossible for them to reproduce a similar level of writing from the ordinary "normal" state. And, of course, what they are experiencing is the truth: the original material is not available to their "normal" focus of awareness.

Something similar happens almost universally to participants in Conferences at Sky Hi Ranch. When they return home, they find it almost impossible to tell other people what has happened to them. In the home "reality," the ranch experience takes on a dreamlike quality. "It was so clear and profound while I was at the ranch," they tell me when they see me later, "but words would dry up in my mouth when I attempted to share what I had experienced." Again we are dealing with state-bound consciousness. While they are at the ranch, Conference participants are not in ordinary states of awareness. Most of these experiences are bound to their levels of consciousness at the ranch and are not fully available to them when they return to the ordinary outer states where most of their friends and family exist. Some participants have actually rejected later what they validly experienced at the ranch. State-bound consciousness also explains the mechanism of the crash or depression that often follows prolonged higher states of experience. The important thing to do in such cases is not to bring the people back to ordinary "reality" but to teach them how to reenter the expanded levels, to recapture and create further on these levels. Again it is all relative because, as you already know, I consider the expanded states of Beingness the natural ones and the "normal" ones profoundly abnormal. The choice of which state to experience life in is always up to the individual.

Invariably one of the participants will say, "I get it, but I want some hope that I can bring it to my everyday life." My response is always the same. It is possible to blend the higher dimensions with the outer levels of awareness, but not if one is unwilling to let go of the rigid structure of that outer everyday life. If one is going to bring experiences through from other levels, one's outer reality must accommodate both. To break free of conditioned states, the belief structure *must* change. If that possibility seems threatening, then one should avoid the pathways into expanded awareness. My clear intention is to break down the partitions that compartmentalize our experience of reality. Your choice is your own.

At the ranch I warn each participant, both in a letter a month before the Conference and in person during the first five days of the Conference, that the exploration of higher states of consciousness can be painful and difficult, like riding a gigantic roller coaster. None of them will return to their homes and professional lives unchanged. Each participant has the choice of remaining or leaving. When the group has committed itself, I begin to intensify the group interaction, and for each individual a window of consciousness begins to open. The participants actually open the window themselves, and near the end of the two weeks, they gradually close the window as they begin to focus their attention on the future event of returning home.

In summary, no creative idea or experience is ever lost: a shift in perspective and state of consciousness only makes it seem to disappear. The practice of meditation teaches us how to change levels of consciousness, so that eventually we can enter any state of consciousness at will, and the creative idea or experience can be fully recovered.

SEQUENTIAL VERSUS SIMULTANEOUS EXPERIENCE

The change of attention toward the return home exemplifies one of the problems of sequential awareness, that of allowing the future — actions that have not yet transpired but are imagined to be going to occur — to influence the present moment. It is the superimposition not of the future but of *ideas* about the future that makes sequential consciousness such a limiting experience. There are many other factors to consider, but this distortion of the experience of the moment is most fundamental.

I believe that the present necessity of communicating by means of words underlies the major entraining of consciousness into sequential linear patterns. Language is indispensable to most human beings — not because it is innate but simply because it is usually the only developed means of communication available to the individual human being. One cannot verbalize two different words simultaneously, and that simple fact is what traps the awareness into sequential patterns. Sequential awareness conditions us in early childhood as we learn to speak, so that the thoughts behind language are trained to appear sequentially in our minds. Soon we begin to experience sequential perception in sight, feeling states and other activities that are not necessarily or inherently sequential at all.

Although most people cannot conceive that it is possible to focus awareness on more than one object or idea simultaneously, some simple training techniques can demonstrate that simultaneous awareness is possible. When simultaneous states of awareness begin to appear, there is an even better alternative to sequentiality — through symbols or through telepathy. Telepathy is capable of impressing in a single moment the *totality* of what is to be communicated.

But communication is just a small part of the insights into the sequential versus the simultaneous. Even though the biochemical reactions at any locus within the brain take place sequentially, thought is not produced by a single biochemical reaction or at a single locus but through the associative reactions taking place simultaneously in many areas of the brain. It is therefore a synthesis of many reactions. I do not wish to imply that thought originates in the brain but only that the brain's physical responses to thought undergo this process. (The late Wilder Penfield of McGill University, Montreal, Canada, a highly respected pioneer in brain surgery, concluded from many years of clinical experience that the human mind cannot be found in the structure of the brain.) Perhaps the brain is a transducer of the basic energy of essential thought, converting this energy or original impress into stepped-down equivalent patterns of energy that the outer mind recognizes as outer or apparent thought. By the time thought appears in the outer awareness, it has been drastically filtered, sequestered and distorted and is of an energy form quite unlike the original.

As I have said before, telepathy is our natural form of communication. Essential thought is not sequential but is an energy configuration that is transformed into a sequential pattern to appear as words or images in the outer awareness. Two people whose outer areas of communication are conditioned to different languages may still be quite capable of communicating with each other — through telepathy. The seeker of another's attention (the "sender") does not have to think in images or symbols, because in telepathy the language is automatically translated into essential thought and retranslated into the outer language of the person having the telepathic impress. Mastery of telepathy would make it possible to abandon language and move to communication by essential thought alone.

So far, I have been using a linear model to discuss aspects of simultaneity. In fact, however, simultaneity has nothing whatsoever to do with linearity or with time. That is, it is neither an affirmation nor a denial of linearity and time; it is simply beyond linearity and time. Time is a useful construct of outer awareness. Essential thought does not know what time is, nor does it care. Essential thought resides in the *now moment*, that all-inclusive dimensionless space of awareness where all of the past, present and future exist simultaneously. I am laughing right now, because it is ridiculously paradoxical to try to use words to discuss nonlinear states, including essential thought.

And I can also laugh at my own experiences as I spent four months of deep contemplation each morning searching for the now moment. The tack that I took was that it was somewhere *between* time and close to the present moment. First I tried to accelerate my awareness into the future slightly to wait for the

now moment to enter my awareness. When that attempt failed
— miserably — I tried to slow time down and escape into the
now moment between time. All I experienced, however, was a
slowed down mind. By then I was exasperated, because I was
sure (erroneously, as I later learned), that *everybody* who taught
higher dimensions of consciousness experienced the now moments. Almost every book on spiritual awareness mentions it. I
felt as if I were some sort of inferior outcast, fenced off in exile
while the superior, acceptable insiders were enjoying the fruits
of the Divine. Then the solution and the experience struck and I
laughed for days. The now moment has absolutely nothing to do
with time. As long as I persisted in trying to reach it through
some alteration of time, I was doomed to failure. The moment I
stopped trying to reach the timeless awareness space and simply
instructed my consciousness to *become* the awareness, it happened. It was an excruciating but important lesson.

In other words, when we talk about the now moment, we
are actually talking about two different things, the present tense,
in which awareness experiences linear, sequential time, and
simultaneity, in which the awareness does *not* experience
linear, sequential time. Both are significant for development.

In Conferences, I use an exercise to demonstrate how little
we are ever aware, in linear time, of the now moment. It is very
simple: for six to eight hours, the Conference participants must
use only the present tense in their conversations with one
another.

Initially I tried the exercise for twenty-four hours, but the
stress on the participants was too great. Six to eight hours is
enough time to demonstrate the experience. Most people try to
get around the frustration by such tricky techniques as using the
present tense to phrase events that really took place in past
moments. Participants discover that it is very hard to talk about
only what is happening in the present moment, especially if
something wonderful happened not long ago (a few minutes to a
few hours) and there was nobody around with whom to share it
as it was happening.

Distorted memories of the past and ideas of the future are

constantly superimposed on the linear now moment. Like pesky flies crawling over one's face, into the nostrils or the mouth, the past and future constantly demand the attention of the focus of our awareness. One can learn finally to ignore all but the present moment. When one does, the opportunity to enter the now moment is available. This is such a supreme state of consciousness to experience that I won't attempt to describe it in words.

Every experience that appears in the outer awareness belongs to the past. Not one iota of that awareness is current. By the time sensory stimuli have been converted from physical energy waves into bioelectrical currents — passed through the brain receivers and translated into coherent images, sounds or feelings, the actual event is over. We are only aware of secondary impressions, not the primary event itself. But in the state of simultaneity, awareness and the events are one and the same. Direct experience is possible, but not through the linear mind patterns. Someday it will be shown that consciousness does not need a physical vehicle to exist. Those people who are capable of moving out of linear patterns already know this to be true, but all the rest — billions of people — do not.

Anything carried over from the past distorts the now moment. There is a story of a man who approached a sage to ask for help with some problems he was having. He had to wait several weeks before he was admitted to the sage's council room, and then the sage only looked at him, asked simply, ''Why are you carrying that huge sack of stones on your back?'' and dismissed him. It took the man several more weeks to understand that the sage's question contained all the insight he needed to solve his problems. That question and that insight are valid for almost everyone.

Past traumas, past hurts, past guilts, past perceptions of reality — especially those of childhood — past beliefs are all stored in the memory mechanism of our consciousness, and we are constantly superimposing them upon our awareness of the moment. If one persists in carrying around the stones of the past, one cannot begin to appreciate the opportunity of a new moment. The heavy, worthless stones of the past must be let go.

One begins by divesting them of any importance. Eventually, because the mind is no longer energizing them, they atrophy: they lose their weight, and there is nothing to carry around anymore.

It is, of course, always appropriate to draw the lesson from the past — what I call "drawing the jewel of insight" — but then, to use a Buddhist expression, the right thing is to *WALK ON!* If you need to punish yourself, carry your stones, but don't then expect to experience any of the other possibilities of life. In ordinary states of consciousness, there simply isn't enough room for both the present and the past.

How is it that the present moment of linear time can be distorted by an event that one expects to occur in the future? What diabolical apparatus of awareness can make us anxious, upset or worried, feel traumatized or sometimes induce illness, with only thoughts about a future event? If you have ever had to prepare for important exams, concert recitals or some other display of talent or knowledge, you know exactly what I mean. Anything, imagined or real, that threatens the ego produces such feelings — until, that is, the ego either dissolves or is deemphasized as the center of one's awareness of self. The actual future event is rarely anything like what you imagine, and the sad part is the squandering of so much energy and the loss of appreciation of the present moments. Only present moments have the potential of being real events and then only if the outer mind doesn't eclipse them.

A wonderful illustration of several of these points is the Old Testament story of Lot and his wife leaving the cities of Sodom and Gomorrah. In metaphysical interpretation, Lot and his wife represent the essential or pure aspects of one's Beingness. Sodom and Gomorrah represent, of course, the distortion and confusion created out of the ignorance of ordinary awareness. The angels that appeared to Lot and his wife symbolize the connection to the higher natural state of Beingness. What did God say to Lot and his wife as they were leaving (the problems, guilts and traumas symbolized by) the city? *Don't look back!*

Don't look back. Extract yourself from these morasses. They have nothing to do with the present moment and certainly not with the future, so long as you, yourself, do not seed the future with the past. Now, what happened to Lot's wife when she did look back? She turned into a pillar of salt; she was rigidified into the form of past actions and past patterns; she was trapped in the past. The injunction is clear: *don't look back,* not even to peek for old time's sake.

Another valid analogy comes from the technique of taking tests effectively in higher education. It usually takes only a few examinations for one to learn not to stop and get bogged down at the first question to which one does not know the answer. What one does instead is to put a check mark by that question and move on through the examination. Often, answers to questions one could not answer are given by later questions, or, as the stress of the examination is discharged and one gets the feeling that most of the questions are answerable, the mind is unblocked and the answer to the difficult question has a chance to come through.

I don't know how many times I have seen individuals, including me, squander an unbelievable amount of time and energy in attempting to cope with a problem. It is a ridiculous situation to sit forever pondering an early question that can't be answered and then to find that the test period is up and you never let yourself go on to other questions that you could have answered easily. The test of Life is analogous. Let go of the problems and get on with living Life. It's a relatively short span of time and not to be wasted on problems—particularly imagined ones! If you come into fulfilling patterns—if you finish the exam before the time period is up—then there is ample opportunity to go back to an old unresolved problem, but, even given that leisure, you do it only if it still appears to be worth the effort.

To get people to let go of their problems is so very difficult. One almost gets the impression that they would be lost without them. If a problem is important to experience, what will appear in the future will not be a specific answer but rather a significant pattern, a template for many similar actions, an overview, which may yield deep insight and wisdom.

Experience the present moments with their potential for an experience of the now moment. Don't look back. Walk on.

BREAKING DOWN THE SKIN-BOUND CONSCIOUSNESS

Many phenomena clearly demonstrate that individuals are not awarenesses residing in the head areas of their physical bodies but are interrelated fields of energy to which the skin presents no barrier at all. Although more and more people are aware of these phenomena and are teaching about them to others, I am often amazed how these people fail to realize the extent to which this knowledge differs from the general consensus of belief of Western humanity as a whole.

If you perform an external-reality check — a check with people who have no idea of reality beyond what is reported to them by their five outer senses and by science in general — you will find that most people consider as sheer nonsense the idea of their Beingness as interpenetrating and coexisting with their physical forms. Healing at a distance, chakra systems, energy fields extending many feet from the surface of the body, telepathy, telekinesis, holographic theory and so on — billions of people do *not* hold these ideas valid. For such people it is a quantum leap in consciousness to find any of these phenomena to be valid by means of an experiential process. There is a vast difference between the mental or intellectual belief that a phenomenon is valid and the direct experience that the phenomenon is valid. The quantum leap occurs only with the experiential route.

As I mentioned earlier, I became extremely interested in the ability to influence other people's energy fields and physical bodies, along with their psychological states, when working at a distance from their bodies. The distance might vary from touching them lightly to working with energy focused through my hands at distances several feet from the body surfaces. Working with someone many miles away is a similar phenomenon, but it requires imaging that person to be in your presence, wherever you and the person may actually be geographically.

We must begin to appreciate the importance of this kind of interaction in relationship to disease—both to its engendering and to its resolution, whether the disease is physical or psychological. A diseased member of a family is not isolated and ineffective in influencing other members of the family, and the other members of the family are involved in influencing the diseased person and his or her disease—*no matter what the disease is*.

The state of consciousness of the people who surround someone who is ill has an influence on the course of the disease in that person. Let me emphasize: I am not talking about *physical* interaction between the people, and I am not talking about the *psychological effects* of words and actions. I am talking about *energy fields*. I am stating that the energy fields of people who surround an ill person—energy fields created primarily out of the unconscious areas of their psyches—can either vitalize the ill person or devitalize the ill person.

People who have strong, healthy bodies and strong senses of well-being radiate this energy without necessarily being aware of what they are doing. In ancient Rome, children were the constant companions, waking and sleeping, of people who were ill; the Romans knew that there was some sort of transfer of vitality from the growing person to the ill one.

Far from being able to modulate their energy fields, most people do not even know they exist. They cannot realize, therefore, the importance of their external attitude and behavior in their relationship to someone who is ill. The energy-field interaction, however, always represents the deeper truth of people's feelings. More than once I have experienced the situation in which a wife professes deep concern for her dying husband while she is also carrying on an extramarital affair; her concern and caring are on the outer levels, but the energy in and attitudes about the affair are deeply involved in her husband's dying—even if he does not know that the affair is going on. In such cases, the field interaction is draining to the patient. The outer mind may be deceived, but the underlying awarenesses of both the patient and the other person react and interact to the truth of what is happening.

Among the people who must be considered in this connection are health practitioners, because they reflect their own state of consciousness and well-beingness as they care for their patients. Tired or upset nurses, physicians, aides, orderlies—anyone, in fact, including the patient in the next bed six feet away—can all influence the sick person in an adverse way. On the other hand, certain physicians, nurses, aides and so on—again including other patients may have naturally uplifting and positive body energies that are conducive to recovery for the patients with whom they come in contact. I remember in particular a nurse's aide from Jamaica: if she simply went in and mopped a sick person's floor, the patient would always report feeling better after she had been in the room. Some nurses—and some doctors—have just the opposite effect. Again, I am not talking about personality differences; I am talking about reflections of deeper consciousness and body energy.

Some day orthodox medicine will recognize that the course of disease is altered by the state of harmony of those who surround and take care of the sick. Health personnel will be taught how to balance their energies and how to share their energies for the benefit of patients. While we now tend to concentrate ill patients in one place, the hospital—which inevitably has a negative field in which it is difficult for the body to recover—we will consider the wisdom of placing a sick person in an environment that is cheerful, without death or serious disease in a bed less than six feet away and surrounded by people who represent health and vitality. Health professionals who are not conducive to a patient's recovery should be removed from the field — or be assigned to people who want to die.

Yes, we must remember that there are situations where vitality and the sense of well-beingness do not serve the patient's purposes. Some patients are preparing for death, and, on the deepest levels, some simply want to die.

When I began my practice of medicine in Los Angeles, I felt an obligation to heal every patient regardless of the cost or the circumstances: it was what my training had taught me. Death was the ogre, the demon to be defeated, and I was the knight dedicated to slaying the dragon. Few patients died while I was on duty. They could die when I was off duty or when a partner was covering my practice, but if a patient—except an aged one—died while I was in charge, I sensed it as a rejection of my skills as a physician. It was a truly difficult experience for me to accept.

This facet of my immaturity was finally shattered by a woman who had been my patient for several years. In her mid-sixties, she suffered from a severe form of heart disease in which the blood vessels to the heart were so constricted that the least exertion or emotional upset was an overload; she sweated profusely, fluid built up in her lungs and she felt excruciating pain in her chest. Once or twice a week for almost a year and a half, most often in the middle of the night, her convalescent home would call me with word that she was in heart failure, with intense pain and marked difficulty in breathing. I would dress and rush to the nursing home, order all the necessary medication and treatments and then go in and give her a pep talk. Within half an hour she would be resting comfortably, and I would leave the nursing home feeling uplifted: I had once more saved the woman's life. What I did not recognize was that, in giving her the pep talk, I was transferring energy to her.

The last time I saw her alive, I had again ordered all the appropriate treatments and she was just coming out of an episode. I was in the middle of giving her my usual encouragement when she suddenly said, "Why are you doing all this to me?" I instantly understood; and I was shocked, then moved to tears. While part of my psyche felt rejection in her words, it was overridden by my deeper sense of compassion and understanding. I stepped out into the hall, where I could openly allow my tears. The woman had confronted me with my fear of facing my own death. In that moment my underlying motivation in "curing" patients and extending myself to keep them from dying was all too clear. I was saving them because I saw them as symbols of me; because I was afraid to die, I was forcing this woman to live—against her will. With this realization I felt a snap inside me, as if some hitherto unknown force field between the woman and me had suddenly been broken. She died within twenty minutes.

Even to this day it is hard for me to keep from transferring vital energy to someone who is dying. Similarly, I often see a family member, or more than one, unknowingly transferring energy and sustaining a dying person, delaying the moment of death. As less myth and greater understanding surround the process of dying, perhaps the dying person will have the strength to die consciously and the members of the family consciously to allow him or her to die. It is only when we comprehend the spiritual or natural states of Beingness that we can begin to understand death.

In this section I also wish to invite my medical peers to reconsider any rigid opinions they may have about unorthodox views on health and disease. Although the principles of orthodox medicine have been, and shall continue to be, basic in our scientific approach to the physical body and in the treatment of emergent or acute disease, much less is understood about the body than is not. Even today many disease processes are simply incomprehensible. Medicine is an art mixed with a great number of hypotheses—about reality, about the human body and about the human mind—and at their deepest levels, most physicians know it.

Altogether, the treatment of disease rests upon empirical experience—essentially trial and error. Hundreds of years of practice have accumulated a body of knowledge that has proved beneficial in alleviating human pain and suffering. The profession is venerated not only because most of its members are dedicated, but also because a person must study and master unbelievable complexities to become qualified as a physician. The medical profession is proud and protective of the standards of practice it has evolved.

As I tell most groups attending Conferences at the ranch, many of them would not be alive to come exploring with me if they had not had the benefits of modern scientific medicine. Some would not have survived the ordinary childhood diseases or other diseases such as pneumonia, which was 50 percent to 80 percent fatal before antibiotics; others would have died of polio, diphtheria or other diseases conquered by orthodox medicine in recent years. For that matter, I wouldn't be there either, because at the age of eighteen months I almost died of double pneumonia. And if you, the reader, advocate natural foods, I must remind you that about two hundred years ago, all our ancestors ate only natural foods, and their average life span was about half what it is today. Natural foods alone will not offer a healthy body. I believe that if you put fine food into a body with a crummy mind, you get a crummy body; but if you put crummy food into a body with expanded awareness, you get a fine body. To a greater extent than we usually realize, our state of consciousness determines the way we transmute the levels of energy represented by foods, but the opposite statement would be definitely untrue: foods do not determine the level of consciousness.

When I practiced orthodox medicine, I was often at the very forefront of knowledge in my attempts to treat the incurable. But my earlier psi abilities, my mother's philosophy and Eunice's demonstrations of healing by mind alone kept coming back to me. I began to feel the need to explore these alternatives in relation to my patients when everything else in the medical armamentarium was failing. Finally my interest broke down my reluctance and my fear.

Through empirical exploration I began to investigate the relationship of the mind to the body. In orthodox medical literature, I studied published accounts of this area of research. I was certain that the mind and body were a unit, and I knew that the idea went back at least as far as Plato and Aristotle. I was also very impressed by cases of "spontaneous remission"— cures partial or complete, temporary or permanent, for no known cause—in patients who had been proved beyond all question to be incurable or terminal. At least in my experience there was, in these cases, usually a spiritual-conversion aspect. Inevitably I became interested in all three areas — spiritual, psychological and physical — and in their interrelationships. I came to lament the peculiar, present-day approach that divided the human being into three separate aspects so that three professions — medicine, psychology-psychiatry and religion — were often needed for a single patient.

In orthodox medical practice, each professional space is jealously guarded, and woe to the person who crosses the line of any of the specialties. To me their boundaries are entirely imaginary; I can't see or feel them. My only concern is to bring to a patient anything and everything to help him or her regain health and a sense of well-beingness. I find that all three areas are involved in every case — and it is as simple as that. Can we also begin to see the analogy of skin-bound consciousness and the compartmentalization of professions?

My intention is to help to break down the irrationally rigid awareness that orthodox medicine displays. I encourage my colleagues to open their minds to new areas of research into the potential of human consciousness and its effects on disease and health. However disturbing these developments may be to medicine's comfortable status quo, it is only a matter of time until medicine recognizes and acknowledges the importance of these fringe areas.

Medicine rests strongly on its foundation, a foundation upon which new advances will arise, beyond the imagination of the most sophisticated practitioners today.

I must emphasize that I am not predicting that the unorthodox approaches will displace medicine. On the contrary, medicine will incorporate some of the so-called unorthodox approaches. Science will demonstrate their validity and give far more insight into bioenergies than any metaphysician has understood to date.

To heal and to alleviate human suffering is the common goal of both the orthodox and the unorthodox practices. The difference between them is simply the difference between their perspectives of reality. Healing does not rest in the hands of a selected few but in the hands of every human being, and I don't mean healing just in the sense of professional therapeutics. I mean that healing can come, will come and does come from the individual integrated human consciousness that is capable of healing itself. No matter what physicians do, they can only augment the healing process of the body itself. The extension of human awareness into the psi areas is only a further diagnostic and therapeutic tool to augment this same basic process.

In August 1974, I discussed these concepts with my medical staff at the hospital with which I was associated. Some of the physicians were shocked, and some were outraged. But, with more and more research material coming out of respected universities, I wonder what their attitudes would be now, just four years later.

I dare to say that the human mind can and does generate force fields that can transmute matter. I further dare to say that an awareness without spiritual foundation is like a stool with only two legs.

THOUGHT FORMS AND ESSENCES

By this time in this book it shouldn't be too difficult to conceive that the human psyche is capable of creating thought forms (forms in thought) that can influence matter, including the physical body. Now I want to talk about the similar process of creating entities — fields of energy that can appear to take on the form of a human, or animal or, for that matter, an angelic being, a demon or even an Inner Teacher.

Whether we are aware of it or not, we are a most wondrous interaction of energy in this dimension and others. Our force fields organize matter into our physical forms. Perhaps an even more essential force field also organizes *subtle matter* into form — that is, the *etheric body*. If you do not know about the aura or the energies that form what is called the etheric body, you may want to read *The Energies of Consciousness*, edited by Stanley Krippner and Daniel Rubin; W.J. Kilner's *The Aura*;

Thelma Moss's *The Probability of the Impossible: Scientific Discoveries and Explorations in the Psychic World; or* William Tiller's section on energy fields and the human body in *Frontiers of Consciousness*, edited by J.W. White.

Occasionally a few people bump into so-called entities — fields of force — that make their presence known through the movement of objects (such as the poltergeist phenomenon), through possession, through spontaneous combustion of materials or through the channeling, during trance or meditation, of what seem to be conscious entities.

If your belief system discounts all such phenomena, you are simply using a convenient way to deal with what is incomprehensible to you. I am impelled to share my own experiences and concepts because this area of exploration is profoundly interesting, and, as expanded awareness begins to be experienced, these phenomena are encountered and must be dealt with. Wait until you experience them! It is in anticipation of that time that I share this information. What I want to do is offset some of the crazy ideas people often have about these manifestations.

I was in my late twenties when such an experience first happened to me. A poltergeist manifestation appeared one evening while I was working on a scientific paper that I was to present to the staff of the Mayo Clinic. I was in the living room of my small, second-story apartment in Rochester, Minnesota, minding my own business, when the hair on the back of my neck suddenly stood straight up. I sensed at once that there was something in the room, but I couldn't see it. Then objects on the kitchen table flew to the floor, and a set of keys on top of the refrigerator catapulted across the room. At this point I could see the vague shape of a vortex of energy moving on the other side of the room. I was so scared that I actually lost control of bowel and bladder. My heart was pounding so hard I thought I was going to have a coronary. If the vortex came any closer to me, I felt, I might die.

Fortunately, there was a phone on the desk. Keeping my eye on the vortex, I carefully picked up the receiver and dialed my mother in Garden Grove, California. I misdialed several times, because I refused to let whatever it was out of my sight. When Mother finally answered the phone, much to my relief, I whispered that there was something in my apartment that wasn't human and felt malevolent. After I told her the events as they had been transpiring, I was shocked by her response.

"Nonsense," she said. "It's only a poltergeist, dear. It won't hurt you if you don't fear it." She sounded almost lighthearted as she said it. "Tell it to go away. Say that it has no business there. Tell it to go back to where it came from."

I felt a calm come over me — then anger. I put the receiver down on the desk top, got up and went over to old whatever-it-was and yelled, "Get out!" Much to my amazement, it did.

Mother laughed when I returned to the phone. "Something in you attracted it," she said. "It's time to see what thoughts inside you attracted it." I didn't fully understand what she meant, but by then it didn't make any difference to me. The thing was gone, and that was all that mattered.

The broken dishes and the keys flying across the room were not in my imagination, nor had I been placing my mind in a suggestible state by reading a ghost story. I was hard at work on a thesis covering a disease related to the pancreas. Even if this event should prove to have been caused by an energy from my own Beingness, it would be awesome; but my feeling is that it was some form of external energy that responded to my telling it to leave.

Several years later, Eunice, during my time of study with her, emphasized the differentiation between thought forms and essences. I, however, paid little attention to this aspect of her work, because to me entities, whether their form was human or demonic, were nothing more than projections of people's minds. Except for my poltergeist experience (which I had by then rationalized as being some natural form of energy vortex not well understood by science) nothing in my experience made me concern myself with the distinctions between thought forms and other supernatural beings or to pay much attention to Eunice's teaching on *protection* and *shielding*.

I can remember her saying that the great deceivers were to be encountered when one entered the subtle levels of awareness. She talked about their presence in the room where she was teaching and about the differences in the kinds of light that emanated from them. "The true spiritual beings of high development have a full aura," she said. "They are filled with a particular quality of white clear light.... Discarnate souls [ordinary people who have died] appear as they did in life, their auric development easy to discern. Thought forms, creatures and forms similar to the human, as well as the demonic, are in the darker shades. Salute the Divinity in them. If they are spiritual beings, they will respond. If they don't, send them on their way." Since I couldn't see any of these entities, or even feel their presence, I would just sit and wait until she discussed areas of more interest to me, such as healing.

In September 1975, I woke one night feeling a powerful presence in my bedroom at the ranch. Its form was human, its colors dark, its feeling demonic. Remembering what my mother and Eunice had said about such things, I simply told it to leave, and it did.

The next morning, in meditation, I asked the Inner Teacher about the presence that had entered my room the night before, and the Inner Teacher delivered a long discourse, of which I remember the essentials:

Just as man is conceived and created out of a higher order of intelligence, so too can man create out of his own order of intelligence. Every time an individual images a person in his or her mind, a *subtle form* of the imaged person is created. Its level of manifestation is ordinarily different from the levels with which we are commonly familiar, but people who are highly developed in the art of thought-form creation can empower their thought forms with enough subtle energy to materialize them. The old-time Tibetans, who were masters of this technique, created many thought forms in the configuration of demons and used them to frighten off unaware humans who might covet things the Tibetans wanted guarded. These thought-form demons were like household pets, often sent to carry out certain missions or, like watchdogs, to ward off enemies. The more demonic-looking the thought form, the more effective it was.

But thought forms aren't restricted to the demonic. Thought forms of saints, Buddha, Christ, wise teachers, angels, gods, animals and so on are all manifested in what is called the astral plane by this mechanism. Once they are created, they remain manifest until a human consciousness dissolves them. If the human who created them dies, the thought forms he or she created remain. From prehistoric times up to the present moment, the human mind has created thought forms for thousands and thousands of years, so that the astral plane is a vast cesspool of these creations, most generated by human consciousness.

The moment human consciousness images, a thought form is created. Most of them, the products of average human minds, have so little substance or intensity as to be of no real consequence. Some, however, are so strong that they can be seen and heard by clairvoyants and other sensitives, and if a thought form is created by many people it is apt to be very powerful. An outstanding and familiar example is the thought form of Christ. Millions of people, imaging the Christ figure, have created millions of thought forms of Christ and have empowered them with all the attributes that human consciousness believes necessary to such a figure. Because of these millions of repetitions, the Christ thought form is a powerful one, and it appears to many sensitives.

Just as we are not consciously aware that we are the creations of a higher order of intelligence, so thought forms do not know that they are thought forms — nor usually, do the psychics who channel them. It is critical to distinguish between the thought form of Jesus Christ, the actual Jesus Christ and the essence of Christ. While the actual Christ exists as a single essence, the Christ thought form exists in unbelievable numbers. The actual Christ essence is not created by the human level of consciousness, but all the others are. In all but rare exceptions, psychics do not bring in the Christ essence; they bring in thought forms of Christ. All thought forms created by the human mind may be dissolved by the human mind, but what the human mind did not create cannot be dissolved by it. This difference can be the key to telling them apart.

The Inner Teacher told me that the entity that had come to me the night before was a thought form that I had created in a previous lifetime. I then asked the Inner Teacher, "How do I know that *you* are not a thought form of mine or someone else's?"

It replied simply, "Try to dissolve me." I couldn't, and, to tell the truth, I didn't especially want to.

The next evening the same negative entity appeared in my room again. It wouldn't leave immediately, and it kept me awake. I felt fear because it was very demonic. Over the next few weeks, it returned every few nights. Finally, in great anger, and with a force I had never before felt pass through my body, I arose from the bed and bellowed an invocation: "I created you, and I now dissolve you!" The demon disappeared and never returned.

People who find themselves doing automatic writing are sometimes channeling thought forms. I know of five different people who believe that they channel the Christ. Of the five, only two are at the level of metaphysical training to be able to distinguish thought form from essence. In such a case, a reading of the material brought through often gives a good idea of whether it is from thought-form area or from the essence.

Several months ago, a gestalt therapist shared with me an interesting phenomenon he had observed when he was working in Brazil. The poorer classes of people there are involved with cults dealing either with black magic — the majority of them — or with white magic. They talk about supernatural entities, demons, good entities and so on. The middle and upper classes who hire the poor as servants, consider such talk sheer superstition and pay it little attention.

Working with a group of middle- and upper-class people in techniques to raise their awareness into transformational states, my therapist friend found, to his amazement, that they were becoming sensitive to thought forms — and they began to report encounters with the thought forms created by their employees!

(The therapist himself had an encounter with some form of energy that pushed him to the ground and forced his head back by pulling his hair.) The lesson here is that disbelief in thought forms seems to have a protective or shielding effect but only so long as people stay away from explorations of subtle reality. If they begin to lose their disbelief, they are unprotected unless they go on through the experience to the start of understanding.

It is a difficult subject, to say the least. What I have said may not be much, but I hope it will be enough to help a beginner, should the need arise.

THE RESOLUTION OF THE DEATH SPACE

Of all the quantum leaps, the resolution of the death space is the most difficult to experience. As we saw in Chapter One, the concept of death is not only encrusted with an overwhelming load of fears, myths, fantasy, ignorance and neurotic ideation, but, also in the West, it is as much as possible shrouded and concealed from experience.

Either physical or psychological death is a transformational experience. (Elisabeth Kübler-Ross puts the idea well in the title of her book, *Death, the Final Stage of Growth*.) No soul that has ever manifested in this plane has escaped it. Nor is it desirable that we should. From the perspective of the unawakened mind, death is such an awesome spectre as to be quickly suppressed or to be discussed in tones that are deadly serious. We may joke about death, but the psychoemotional reaction to the actual event, whether the death of loved ones or the knowledge of the approach of one's own death, is probably the most profound experience ordinary consciousness must meet. The end of the physical self, or the threatened end of the psychological self, is one of the central fears of the human being. It demonstrates our usual identification of the aware state of consciousness with the outer manifest plane, with the body and the ego or personality level. When one is able to break free of this identification, when one knows experientially that body and ego are not the sole totality of one's Beingness, the transformational states of consciousness can become available while one is still embodied.

It took me a long time to catch a glimpse of a higher self beyond the ego level. I had plenty of ideas about such a self but had no real experience of it until I committed myself to the deidentification with the ego, to embrace what I call the Higher Orchestrator. I spent nine months working on the death process in terms of the ego or ideas about myself. During that time I became aware that I would also have to deidentify with my body. In other words, the fear of physical death and psychological death would have to be released, and the only way I knew to do it was to trust that my Beingness was more than either my body or my ego. That trust was based on rare and brief experiences through meditation.

Please note carefully that I am not speaking about destroying the physical form or the ego. I am speaking about the expansion into a state of awareness where the loss of either is of no importance. This state is immortality, and it has absolutely no concept of death. Literally, it does not know that death exists, because, deathless itself, it experiences bodies and personalities only as vehicles to express itself. It is the outer mind that creates the pain surrounding death, because death itself is only a marker, or gate, that signals to the deeper awareness that a lifetime is now complete. Because of the continuity of Beingness, the deep awareness does not even experience the actual moment of death.

I have enjoyed Edgar Cayce's comments on this subject. He said in one of his readings that if only the outer awareness knew the fear and apprehension of the soul just *before* incarnating into the plane, there would be far less fear about passing out of it.

The greatest psychological pain of the death process is caused by the attachment to the form nature, whether it be to other people, one's own body, places, whatever. To conquer this pain and the fear associated with it, detachment must be achieved.

To psychologists and psychiatrists, detachment is a

symptom of an abnormal state of consciousness. If the detachment is complete, it is called a psychotic break, a loss of connection with reality. I want to emphasize clearly that I am not discussing a state of consciousness that is disconnected from reality; I am discussing a state of consciousness that is aware of ordinary reality but is also aware of an even higher portion of Beingness. In this state, one does not overvalue either the ego or the body, because neither is essential to the existence of the higher consciousness.

A psychotic break is, however, a genuine risk in the practice of detachment. Unless one has at least a thin thread to guide the awareness to the higher levels, the mind can lose itself in universes that have no connection at all to outer reality. There is a slight risk on the return to the usual perspective of outer reality, but it is nothing in comparison to the risk involved in releasing ego boundaries to embrace the higher self. This risk is especially great if one has a tendency to reject either the self or the outer reality. Detachment and rejection lead to quite different consequences. While detachment has the potential of enlightenment, rejection has the potential of neurosis, of psychosis, of death of the physical body or all three. Detachment produces the serenity of releasing to embrace, while rejection produces anguish, pain and let-me-out-of-here feelings.

As a preparation for this detachment without rejection, contemplation on the *Tibetan Book of the Dead* and the *Egyptian Book of the Dead* can be extremely helpful. They can also be terribly confusing, if one doesn't catch the essentials. In the process of detachment come fifty-six demons, and each one of them represents individual or collective fears that can deflect the soul from the straight path and completely block its progress if the awareness gives them even the slightest acknowledgment. The fifty-six demons must simply be ignored.

I reached the culmination of my work on the process of psychological death with my experience in the Great Pyramid of Cheops. Before I relate that experience, I will explain how I managed to arrange to spend the night alone in the Great Pyramid.

I went to Egypt from Findhorn with two wonderful friends, David Elliott and Pat MacLean. I had three objectives in mind. One was to scan the mummies in the Cairo Museum. (I'll discuss scanning in the next chapter.) Another was to visit the Karnak ruins. The last was to spend a night alone in the Great Pyramid.

On arriving in Cairo, we headed straight for the pyramid and took the usual guided tour through it. It was amazing to me, because while the pyramid is huge, the passageways up to the grand gallery and into the queen's and king's chambers are so small that one can only crawl or waddle to get through them. On entering the grand gallery, one has to climb a series of steel rungs to reach a walkway that, in turn, ascends to the entrance of the king's chamber. Some major drop-offs have no railing for protection. On the guided tour, I made a mental map of the pyramid in preparation for my solitary adventure.

Outside the pyramid, one of the tour guides asked whether I wanted to spend some time alone inside. From stories I had heard, I guessed it was going to cost some money to make arrangements, so I went to work on my best business and bartering states of consciousness. I might be interested, I said, but it would have to be for the entire night of the full moon, two days away, and I needed to be entirely alone. "Hmmmmm, this is very difficult," the guide responded, and I began to see the dollar signs go up in brilliant neon, rising higher and higher into the sky. I agreed to meet him the next day for a report on his progress in getting me in.

Since it was still early afternoon, Pat, David and I decided to climb to the top of the pyramid to meditate on the setting sun. Our plan was to assault the top by going straight up the north face. About a third of the way up I realized that it was a crazy thing to do. The face of the pyramid had been eroded by centuries of wind-driven sand, so that handholds and footholds could crumble or break off at a touch. It didn't seem to bother David; he had nearly reached the top.

I experienced several minutes of panic. I was about two hundred feet up and wasn't really sure I could get down. When I looked down, there were all these people screaming up at me in Arabic. When I did get down, an Arab who spoke English told me that the way I had been going was the most difficult way to climb the pyramid and that, in fact, at least nine people a year are killed trying it. "I'll show you the way," he said. It didn't cost as much as I thought it would.

The pyramid is more than 450 feet high, with an angle of incline of $51^0, 51'$. The corner edges are huge blocks, like giant steps, and so I climbed up them until I was about two-thirds of the way up. At that point, I was startled by a tremendously powerful urge to cast myself off. Never in my life had I experienced such an impulse. Instead of lessening, it intensified as I continued upward, and I had to use every last degree of control not to jump. The moment I reached the apex, however, the feeling dissipated. The experience was eerie, almost as if there were some sort of barrier or force field one had to pass through. Later, I climbed the pyramid several times without sensing the barrier field, but that first blast was almost too much for me.

The next day the guide informed me that it would not be possible to stay in the pyramid overnight. *More money,* I thought. Finally, I politely asked him who was in charge of the pyramid. "A professor of Egyptian antiquities over there," he said, pointing to some sand dunes.

"I'll talk to him," I replied. So I went over the sand dunes, found the small, adobelike structure with its office, and encountered the official, a young man who spoke excellent English and was shrewd. When I told him I would like to spend some time alone in prayer in the pyramid, he seemed perfectly agreeable and offered to arrange for a three-hour period late that afternoon, after the pyramid was closed to the public. When I told him I wanted to spend the entire night alone inside the pyramid, his attitude changed. Before I realized what was happening, I found myself undergoing another psychiatric interview — one of several I endured in 1975.

I convinced him I was sane, and that my motives were coherent. (I was deliberately a little misleading. How could I tell him I was working on the death process and detachment?)

He informed me that only the president of Egypt could give permission for me to stay in the pyramid for the entire night. What the young official could arrange was for me to be inside from five to eight that evening after the pyramid had closed to the public, and again from five to eight in the morning, before it opened. I immediately saw how I was going to spend the whole night in the pyramid, and asked him if I could accept his offer of time alone in the pyramid for the next evening.

He agreed, but also delivered a warning about a long stay in the pyramids. "Too many people become psychotic if they spend more than just a few hours at a time in there" was the last thing he said to me.

Promptly at 5:00 P.M. on the night of the full moon in February 1975, I met the gatekeeper who was to let me in and take me out at the appropriate time. A payment of fifteen Egyptian pounds to the gatekeeper enabled him to forget to let me out that evening.

The gate was locked behind me as I began my penetration to the first inclined tunnel. It was dark and cool. 5:10 P.M. Full moon.

When I entered the pyramid to spend the night, I was free to release the world, my form and my ego. I had already detached myself from everything and everyone else. The most difficult detachment for me to achieve had been from my two brothers, especially my twin. One would have thought it would be my mother or my father, but it wasn't. The release of my twin brother had been almost unbearable. It had taken place an hour earlier in a meditation between the paws of the Sphynx.

I felt fear of psychosis, but only momentarily. I was aware of something else inside me guiding this initiation, as if I had experienced it all before in other lifetimes — an Egyptian lifetime, a Tibetan lifetime, a Zen-Buddhist lifetime and a Christian monk lifetime. Even the demonic thought forms that greeted me on my entrance turned out to be old, familiar, almost friendly experiences.

I was not, however, in such a state of consciousness as to be entirely free from childhood memories of such horror movies as *The Mummy's Curse* and its sequel, *The Return of the Mummy*. As I said earlier, the usual work with thought forms is merely to ignore demons, but there was also another effective maneuver—to laugh at them. Laughter turned out to be the most effective way to dispel them.

When the demons disappeared, I felt a tremendous sense of freedom. Now I had access not only to the deepest aspects of the pyramid, but to the deepest aspects of my own Beingness as well. My eyelids seemed like cellophane, because I could not tell whether my eyes were open or closed. When I paused before the entrance to the first small passage, I began to notice a light that seemed to touch my body and to extend for several feet. At first I suspected that I might be hallucinating, but as I inched my way along the walls, what I felt with my hands correlated with what I was seeing. My ego boundaries were dissolving, and the pyramid and I were fusing into a unit. I spent almost three hours in the queen's chamber, then ascended to the king's chamber for nine hours of experiences beyond my ability to articulate even today.

After twelve hours, the process of detachment and expansion ended. I had died in those twelve hours. Whatever configurated my consciousness as William Brugh Joy, M.D., was gone. I was an incarnation of another aspect of my Beingness in the same physical vehicle. It would take several years for it to mature, but my consciousness had been fully impregnated with information and I had completed the experience of entering states of awareness I had not even dreamed of. I was ready to begin the journey back down.

I reached the opening of the pyramid at 6:10 — the approach of sunrise. As if by magic the gatekeeper appeared and unlocked the gate. I felt something even greater than exhilaration. It was ananda! I climbed the pyramid to experience the sunrise and the full moonset.

It was rebirth.

My encounter with inner death was completed, but my outer death work was not. In Auroville, India, a month after my night in the Great Pyramid, I suddenly decided to return to the United States. My outer reason was my desire to complete the ceremony of becoming a Fellow of the American College of Physicians. I could have chosen to do it the following year, and I was experiencing an almost incredible state of integration and well-beingness in India, but the pull back to the United States was the force that determined my action then.

After I was confirmed as a Fellow—in San Franciso on April 7, 1975—I traveled down the coast of California, took a side trip to the desert to spend a few days at the ranch and reached Los Angeles on the morning of the 17th of April. I was visiting a friend when Father telephoned. My mother, who had previously enjoyed perfect health, had collapsed. The rescue squad was attempting cardiac resuscitation.

I went into a deep meditation, and my mother spoke to me. She said that she was going to die but would not leave her body until I was with her at the hospital, forty-five minutes away. In the emergency room, I talked briefly with the physician in charge. "She is stable but comatose," he said.

I pulled back the white curtain that surrounded her. She was on a respirator, and two IVs were running. Electrocardiographic electrodes were on her arms, on her left leg and over her heart. The monitor showed the heart to be regular in rhythm but acutely injured. I scanned her energy field quickly, then went to the heart area and began to transfer energy to her. It was like a steel wall. Not one speck of energy would move into her body. I went to the head area and tried again. Again there was no transfer of energy. Her eyes were dilated. She was serene and strikingly beautiful, like a Nefertiti. Five minutes after I had arrived, her heart stopped. No medication, no countershock, nothing could stimulate it into activity. She was gone. I removed her wedding ring and turned to cry. A nurse who was working beside me held me for those moments of pain and tears as the physical bonding between mother and son was broken.

In a two-week Conference at the ranch, two days are set aside to explore the spaces of the now moment, death and transformation or reincarnating with new vision. This period — actually nearly sixty hours — combines fasting with total silence. One has the opportunity to enter the desert in solitude. The participants examine what each one would change in his or her life if this experience were to be an actual death. What attachments would pull one back for another lifetime? How does hanging on to problem areas make it necessary, in the future of this lifetime and in future lifetimes, to continue the manifestation of such problems? What overview or vision of totality of Beingness can be glimpsed and experienced? Can we release our identification with the body and personality level and embrace a higher authority of our Beingness? What is Unconditional Love and how is it expressed?

The two days are agony and ecstasy, a battle for mastery over self.

THE EXPERIENCE OF UNCONDITIONAL LOVE

The importance of Unconditional Love was so obvious to my awareness, I had felt no need to include it, separately and specifically, in any of my public or private discussions focused upon quantum leaps in consciousness. Then, earlier this year, a Conference participant asked me to choose which of the transformational shifts I considered most important in my experiences up to that moment. It was only then that I realized the gross omission. Unconditional Love is the most fundamental and transforming of all the leaps. It is mentioned with emphasis in numerous places in this book, but, most important, it is the field force that penetrates all of the book, of my work and of my life.

To use the terminology of ancient Greece, Unconditional Love is most closely equated with Philos, or brotherly love, and is beautifully poised between Eros, which is sexual-emotional love, and Agape, which is purely spiritual love. While Agape tends to exclude the form nature, Eros tends to exclude the spiritual aspects. Unconditional Love synthesizes Agape and Eros.

Without the opening into Unconditional Love, as manifested by the opening of the heart chakra, the states of awareness achieved through the opening of the higher chakras cannot be integrated with those of the lower chakras. Unconditional Love connects the body to the soul.

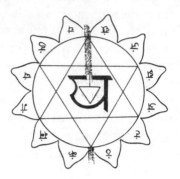

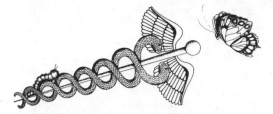

CHAPTER SEVEN

Command Therapy, the Chakras, Body Scanning, Energy Transfer, Healing

You are not inside your body; your body is inside you.

In meditation in the spring of 1973, I had several dialogues with the Inner Teacher on the subject of visualization and the mechanism by which an aspect of thought is able to materialize matter and cause events. During one of these dialogues, I suddenly perceived, all at once, the six steps of a visualization technique to use in healing. I named it Command Therapy and saw it as a powerful tool that patients could use for themselves in the healing of their own bodies.

Mental imagery is the basis of mental healing. Its mastery is fundamental to all the ancient mystery schools and to Hermetic teaching. It is the central technique used by Christian Science, Religious Science, Science of Mind and all other organizations, whether religious, metaphysical or simply practical, that profess or practice the power of mind over matter.

Visualization requires exquisite control over the portion of

145

the mind that has the power to create objects, ideas and events. In the human consciousness, it is an inheritance that few claim and even fewer have mastered. That it works is undeniable. How it works can only be hypothesized.

Eunice was a mistress of the visualization technique. Her power to create an image in extreme detail was formidable. "The outer mind must be made to function as you wish it to function," were her exact words, and she taught a meditation technique that specifically developed this faculty. Once one had reached a relaxed, quiet state of mind, one was to image a large black curtain on which one was to begin the process of pinning up numbers one by one, from one to one hundred. The numbers were to be large, golden in color and perfect. They could not be hazy nor could they waver. One could not take down a number until it had been on the black curtain in clear detail and bright color for at least five seconds. Note that the numbers did not just appear on and disappear from the screen; Eunice had the individual pin up and take down each number. The difference was important, because in her teaching the process was to be identified with self-mastery. The hands that pinned up the number and the pin used to hang the number on the curtain must be seen as clearly as the numbers themselves. Simple though it may sound, the mastering of this technique is not easy. For me, it took many weeks to get the numbers to stay focused, many more weeks to keep them from floating off the black curtain. From my experiences, however, I know it is worth the effort. Not only does it sharpen the visualizing mechanism of the mind, but also it heightens one's ability to call up, at will, during meditation, an entire dream from just a fragment remembered by the outer mind. In addition, it vastly strengthens the power of concentration.

Note the difference between this disciplined approach, where one creates precisely what one wishes, and the free-imagery approach, where the mind wanders and creates whatever images it wants while the individual is simply an observer. One is active and directive, while the other is passive and permissive. (The passive technique is used therapeutically in the form of guided imagery, to allow subconscious ideation and patterns to appear in the outer awareness as images reflecting an experience that the client "imagines." The therapist then guides the client into imaging the resolution to whatever problems came up in the initial images. This passive technique is invaluable in detecting underlying fears, motivations and fantasies that are influencing the client's experience of the outer reality.) Both techniques, the disciplined-willed and the passive-allowing, function to alter the manifest plane through the principle that thought and matter are functionally related.

Einstein's genius demonstrated this principle beautifully with his famous equation $E = mc^2$. If the equation is rearranged, by simple algebra, we can see the relationships differently: $c^2 = \dfrac{E}{m}$. Really feel into what this equation is expressing! Energy and mass, always in the same proportion, are equated with the square of a constant numerical value for the speed of light.

A metaphysical interpretation of this equation would designate c^2 as equivalent to consciousness, and mass and energy as its aspects. Thought is a form of energy, and its complementary manifestation is mass. The equation also says that there is an enormous amount of energy in proportion to whatever mass is present, no matter whether we are talking about an atom or about a universe. Since energy and mass are always in the same ratio, addition of energy to a system means that its mass must increase — and if mass is added, energy must increase tremendously. Can we begin to see the meaning of earlier statements that we are primarily energy and only a tiny bit mass? Compared with the mass of our Beingness, the energy is beyond the imagination of the outer mind!

Mathematics is not a reality in itself but a language that describes experiential reality. The fact that c^2 is a constant and that the ratio between E and m is constant, implies *law* underlying the manifestation and interaction of energy and mass. In essence, consciousness does not care about quantity, only about proportion or balance. There are other, deeper relationships hidden in this simple equation, but these few should send you on into an exciting contemplation.

According to another hypothesis, unconnected to Einstein's equation, matter is present or manifest (like an electric light turned on) for only a brief part of any given moment and not manifest (turned off) for most of any given moment. In other words, manifest reality is both here and not here (on and off) but mostly not here (off). Since your physical body is matter, it too is not here most of the time.

Because our awareness perceives only the "on" parts of the moments, we simply cannot appreciate the ones that are "off." In the same way, our eyes are not aware of the "off" moments between the frames of a motion-picture film. In movies we see 24 separate pictures (frames) per second. The rapid sequence not only produces the illusion of motion but also makes possible so-called subliminal advertising, in which one or several frames per second, instead of being part of the picture sequence, can be used to flash product images or other selling symbols. The outer mind can't see them, but the "unaware" portion of the subconscious does see them and responds to them. Subliminal advertising works — works so well that it has been legally banned — and its success clearly indicates that some part of the consciousness is working and perceiving even when the outer mind is not. With some rather elaborate technology, using two synchronized projectors, it might be possible to show two or more movies at the same time, one being the regular film, with the others being subliminal features shown during the intervals when the screen was dark between the frames of the regular film.

It is easy to see why subliminal advertising has been banned. But almost all forms of advertising and propaganda take advantage of subliminal influence. If we were fully aware of how we are manipulated subliminally, most of us would be outraged. The fault is ours. We choose to be ignorant of these influences. What we are aware of doesn't seem to bother us even though we are literally unaware of most events taking place in ordinary reality! Subliminal forces also exist in other areas. They raise the frightening prospects of psychic warfare and political manipulation. Only time can tell us how significant these forces will be in the course of human events.

The human energy field is capable of converting matter into energy and energy into matter. This fundamental principle enables the visualizing technique to work in cases of physical transmutation, materialization and dematerialization. Scientifically inclined people may object that the energies released by, or required for, the interchange of energy and matter are tremendous — as in nuclear weapons — but, somehow, in a currently unexplained manner, it is possible to buffer or to catalyze the interchange between matter and energy without the uncontrolled violence that conventional science knows.

As science comes to study the phenomena of materialization and dematerialization, cold light, bioluminescence, the body's ability to transmute various atoms into other atoms and such other force-field behavior as instantaneous healing — all areas incomprehensible in current scientific theory — there will be less squabbling and greater insight into the fabulous power of the mind. The modulating mechanism is there; all we have to do is discover it.

I believe that the human body is an outrageously ingenious demonstration of the power of consciousness to turn energy into matter and matter into energy. With this insight we can now undefine ourselves and stop defining our limitations. No matter how far advanced science may be, its compendium of knowledge is only in its infancy compared to all the still undiscovered knowledge that the physical body-mind interactions have to teach.

The body is a natural transmuter. It is the Philosopher's Stone, capable of converting other forms of energy and matter into itself. If you don't quite believe this, pause for a moment and try to comprehend how the body is turning that leaf of lettuce into an eyeball, or that chicken or piece of cow into you. It is not quite within the conceptual framework of science, but the body is potentially capable of turning anything into itself. The human body is also a simple demonstration that it takes life form to sustain life form in more highly evolved species in the manifest plane.

But the body also has the ability to tap alternative or latent sources of energy, other than food, in order to manifest itself. There are documented cases of individuals who have sustained themselves on nothing but rare sips of water, or sips of water and occasional Communion wafers, for years on end.

The body-mind organization is positioned, between matter and nonmatter, precisely at the interface between the manifest plane and all other dimensions. Just as the eye cannot see itself, the perceiving mechanism of consciousness cannot see this interface. Here, where our physical and mental Beingness meet, energies from other dimensions, and not just the energy sources currently known, are available to manifest our Beingness. Essential thought is just one example of an energy from sources not of this dimension. In fact, the vaster portion of our Beingness is not in this dimension.

The easiest, most rudimentary way to reach understanding of this conceptual framework is visualization. And so we arrive back at Command Therapy, and its exploration, as a preliminary to the discovery of the body-energy fields.

Step One in Command Therapy is to relax as completely as possible. Many books describe relaxation techniques in detail. People differ as to the techniques they find effective. Whatever works for you is fine. One technique I like is to imagine that you are a chunk of butter melting under the warmth of the noonday sun. Allow your body to "melt" into relaxation. By the time you feel that you have become liquid butter, the relaxation process should be complete.

In the end, all tension in the body must be released. One should *feel* the body to be relaxed and not just imagine it. Without going to sleep, really let go into the relaxation process. (Studies on muscle relaxation have shown that anxiety is not a feeling state produced by the psyche but a product of muscular tension. It is impossible to feel anxiety if your body is totally relaxed). Soft, gentle music is helpful, and so is a warm room. (Eventually the relaxation process can take place in the most chaotic circumstances; but for the beginner, a comfortably warm, quiet room is the place to start.) If during the relaxation process some part of the body begins to tense, pay attention. Identifying areas difficult to relax will help you see where you carry most of the tension in your body, and this understanding may lead to deeper psychological insights. Most people carry tension in the pelvic area, shoulders, hands, arms and neck. If you feel pain in this process, don't resist it. Relax into the painful area. Simply allow it to be present, without concerning yourself with it. If you do not try to push it away, it will not push back, and you may find that it diminishes by itself.

Step Two requires that you recapture a memory of an inspirational experience. In this way you begin to entrain the emotional and feeling areas of consciousness to flood the body with a sense of well-beingness. You also shift the perspective of your awareness from thinking of your medical problem to a frame of mind where you naturally and spontaneously envision health and a sense of vitality.

Many reports in the medical and psychological literature show the destructive action of stress, depression, unhappiness or fatigue on the body. One of the physiological responses is a weakening of the body's natural defense mechanism, a portion of which is the immune reaction, the activity of the white blood cells and the antibodies. The major thrust of science till now has focused on bacteria, viruses and other microorganisms as the causative agents in many diseases. I do not mean to call them unimportant — but far more fascinating to my mind are the mechanisms of the body itself that let these organisms penetrate the defenses and establish disease. Every person carries on or in the body organisms that are capable of producing serious disease; but most diseases, most of the time, simply do not appear. In the disease process, the decline of the immune mechanism is one major factor, and it is clearly influenced by negative psychological attitudes or feeling states. Becoming overtired from self-imposed long work schedules, worry and stress over "problems" and so on reduces the body's ability to withstand invasion and accelerates the wear and tear responses in the body. One's resistance is reduced, not just to infection but to a host of such other diseases as coronary-artery disease, peptic ulcers, diabetes mellitus — diseases in which invading organisms are not a factor. To my mind, therefore, the sense of well-being and relaxation might have the effect of increasing the body's defenses and sense of integration — breaking up the vicious cycles induced by psychological and physical stress and fatigue states. My hypothesis is that a sense of well-beingness might even stimulate the immune mechanism (and presumably other factors as yet undiscovered) to help the body eliminate *any* disease process.

Although cancer is not considered a bacteria-caused disease, the value of antibodies and white blood cells in its treatment is well-known. One technique, in fact, uses BCG, an agent derived from the organism that causes one kind of tuberculosis to stimulate the patient's immune system to fight the cancer. The patient doesn't develop tuberculosis, but rather the great stimulation of the immune mechanism causes the production of agents that are able to work against the cancer.

One current theory in cancer treatment is that if the cancer cells are reduced to a certain critical (but undefined) number, the body's own natural immunity (if still intact) will take care of the rest. Science is quite certain that cancer cells develop daily in every person's body and believes that the body's natural immunity eliminates these malignant cells daily. If the immune mechanism of the body is depressed, however, the chances of cancer (and for that matter, many other diseases) are increased. Though I must caution you that the immune mechanism is not the only factor to consider in cancer and disease in general, it is an important one and, since the psychological attitude of the patient can either augment or depress the healing of the body, love, happiness, inspiration and a sense of fulfillment are keys to invoking well-beingness. So, in this step, we are using a positive attribute of the memory — that of guiding the awareness to the memory of a past event that was uplifting and harmonious.

Step Three is to make all the feeling sensations of that inspiring memory present in the body while doing this technique. Through the memory we guide the awareness into that space or perspective in consciousness that produces a sense of well-beingness in the present moment. This step is critical, because simply remaining in a memory of a past event does no good. It is not enough. The memory must be transposed to the present moment, and its feeling tones in the body must be fully activated. Here we are taking advantage of both the power of mental imagery and the power of the emotional system. When the emotional feeling tones are combined with imagery, the overall response is greatly intensified.

Step Four is to know that this feeling and this state of consciousness are supportive to the healing process of the body. Feel it counteract the disease or stimulate the healing of any problem in the body. Focus the sense of well-beingness directly into the problem area or areas. Don't *think* that it is doing this. *Feel* it! Even if you are not consciously aware of where all of the disease process is in your body, something in your consciousness does know. Trust that your consciousness will carry this healing sensation to every cell of your body that is not healthy and vital.

Step Five is to visualize the disease actually improving, becoming less and less intense and finally being replaced by normal healthy tissue. Don't worry how this process is to be accomplished. The body knows how to eliminate disease, even if your conscious awareness does not. The work of your conscious awareness is just to see and feel the disease disappearing and to see and feel healthy tissue filling in where the disease was. Talk to your body, explain that you are willing to do anything that is needed to help it recover, and it will cure itself. Your body will cure you!

The Sixth (and last) Step is to visualize yourself as perfectly well and engaged in a future activity. Consciously use great detail in this last visualization. See your friends, your family, your spouse — everybody — all responding to how wonderful you look. Feel your sense of well-beingness and excitement over your total recovery from the illness. Feel your body walking, running, dancing, swimming, playing golf — whatever. Really get into it. Conclude this exercise with a deep sense of your wholeness: you are spiritually connected, psychologically harmonized and physically well.

While you are going through the experience of Command Therapy, keep in mind that science and medicine do not know all there is to know about the healing process. However much is definitively known, there always remains a big X factor. The body always has many additional, wondrous ways to heal.

During the initial stages of Command Therapy, whether or not you are using it in conjunction with conventional therapy, the six steps of visualization should be practiced three times a day — upon first waking, at midday, and shortly before retiring. As the disease begins to remit, Command Therapy can be reduced to a morning exercise. Eventually you will find that a morning exercise of simply establishing a sense of well-beingness is more than ample.

The process of visualization can be fatiguing. The last three steps — especially the final one — must be accomplished with the same enthusiasm and energy as the first three. It is important, therefore, that you learn to pace yourself through the exercise. If you become fatigued initially, start out more slowly and easily the next time. ABOVE ALL, ENJOY THE EXERCISE!

I feel strongly that the disease process itself should not be visualized in detail and with great mental effort, for the laws behind visualization can operate as strongly to configurate disease as they can to dissolve it. For the same reason, do not keep visualizing the disease as it was when you began Command Therapy. Keep your visualization up to the minute. See or feel it as it is currently manifesting in the body at the beginning of *each* repetition of the exercise. Above all, don't worry about whether you are doing it right. There is a magnificent trust that develops between your participation in your own healing process and all other modalities being brought to the body for its cure. Surrender into the process.

For the cancer patient, Command Therapy can be used to augment chemotherapy and radiation therapy. To Steps Three and Four, add the taking into the body of these healing agents, and mentally direct the agents to the diseased areas. Feel and see the chemical or radiation destroying the disease process. Command your consciousness that you want *no* side effects from these therapies, nothing but the body reactions that will heal the disease. Very often the patient's own deep psychological resistance to therapy impairs the functioning of chemotherapy and radiation. Now you can open fully to the treatment because you can *command* the body to display no side effects. You must evoke will in this action. Many patients with whom I used Command Therapy consistently required less chemotherapy and less intense radiation — and both for shorter periods of time. Tell your therapist that you are working on treatment in this manner, or else overdosage of radiation or chemotherapy is possible.

The same concept holds true when any medication is taken into the body. Clear away your resistances and prepare your body to receive the medication. Allopathic drugs are powerful, but not as powerful as the integrated human being. You can modulate the radiation passing into your body, as well as the action of any form of medication.

My discovery of energy fields radiating from the body surface, like my discovery of the principles of Command Therapy, occurred in 1973 — and quite by accident. Since Eunice's death, late in 1972, my only teacher was the Inner Teacher, with whom I was in daily contact in morning meditation.

One day in my office I was examining a healthy male in his early twenties. He was quietly lying on the examining table. I finished listening to his heart and lungs and was approaching the examination of the abdomen. As I was feeling for the edge of the liver, just under the right lower rib cage, I felt a strange impulse to see whether I could detect energy radiating from the liver. It is a large organ and metabolically very active, with high internal temperatures. I lifted my right hand approximately six inches from the body surface and began to pass it over the liver area. I half expected to feel a slight warmth, but I felt absolutely nothing. Then, as my hand passed over the solar plexus area, the pit of the stomach, I sensed something that felt like a warm cloud. It seemed to radiate out three to four feet from the body, perpendicular to the surface and to be shaped like a cylinder about four inches in diameter.

I was astonished! In the first place, there was no organ system in the area that could radiate such a field of energy. True, the liver crosses the midline and extends to the left side of the upper abdomen, but if this radiation of energy came from that small part of the liver, why didn't the major portion of the liver radiate it, too? I simply had no idea what I was feeling. Fortunately for me, the patient's eyes were shut, because there I was with my eyes closed, passing my hand back and forth over his upper abdomen, sometimes as far as five feet away from his body, making sure that what I felt wasn't the product of my imagination. Each time I crossed over the solar plexus area, I felt the same energy field. As I concluded the examination, I made a mental note to discuss the incident with the Inner Teacher the next morning.

The Inner Teacher simply said, "There are other areas of the body that radiate similar fields. Map them." Fine. It was much easier said than done. What would my patients think if they saw me passing my hand over their bodies in this way? So I asked my patients to close their eyes and to relax while I examined them; and I quickly, silently felt for radiation over each area I had routinely examined in the orthodox fashion. At first, if patients opened their eyes to say something and found me off in space with my eyes closed, moving my hands back and forth at some distance above the body, I was embarrassed; but I learned to cover myself casually by saying that heat can sometimes be felt at a distance from the body, and I was checking for it. I usually got away with it, but occasionally a patient would

ask, "Are you one of those doctors who practices magic?"
Some questions were even harder to evade, and it was particularly embarrassing if a nurse or a fellow physician walked in the
room while I was doing my "magic."

During the first three months I did not know what I was
feeling or what the implications of the fields were, but gradually
a pattern began to emerge. Everybody I "scanned" (the word I
use for this aspect of body-field work) had several cylinderlike
radiations coming from the body — off the top of the head; from
the forehead just above the roof of the nose; from the center of
the throat just above the junction of the collar bones; from the
center of the upper chest, about a third of the way down from the
neck; from the center of the chest, about two-thirds of the way
down from the neck; from the solar plexus, the pit of the
stomach; off the left upper abdomen, the area of the spleen;
from the center of the lower abdomen, just above the pubic
bone; from the area just above the genitals; from both the knees
and from the toes and the fingers. (See Figs. 7.1—7.5, pgs.
167-171.)

I mapped out these energy fields during the first three
months. They were present to a greater or lesser degree on each
person I examined. They were detectable anywhere from a few
inches to as far as six feet away from the body surface. To me,
they always felt like a warm, subtle sensation to my hands. For
these first explorations, I was indeed fortunate to have mostly
healthy persons who were there only for their annual physical
examinations, because I did not yet know that localized diseases
radiate similar fields of similar intensity. That part of the exploration was to come during the next three months of study.

From this description some readers will already know
exactly what the distribution of the energy areas of the body
reflected. Please realize that I was so innocent of such matters
that I had no idea what the pattern meant. Then one day,
browsing in the Bodhi Tree bookstore in Los Angeles, I happened to see a book on Tantra Yoga. It was opened to a drawing
several thousand years old, that showed many circular areas
marked on the body surface of a person who appeared to be in

deep meditation. Most of these circled areas corresponded to the areas that I had been mapping. According to the book, they were called chakras, and their interrelationships formed the chakra system. The Bodhi Tree is ordinarily quiet and serene, but not in that moment. "My God!" I exclaimed aloud. "I have discovered the chakras!" And so I had.

Chakra is a Sanskrit word meaning "wheel." The wheel is the disk or wheel of rotating energy that some clairvoyants can see in the major chakra areas of the body. It appears to be just above or below the body surface, and each chakra is conventionally distinguished by the color or colors composing its rotating disc. In yoga, the activation and development of the chakra system is the pathway to illumination, because each chakra — running from the root (at the perineum) to the crown (at the top of the head) — confers its individual powers and states of awareness.

One surprise that I had was that no books I could find showed something that I had observed — that the chakras radiate a field of energy that extends, in some people, as far as twenty feet away from the body.

Also, since I could not see the chakras at that time, the references to colors made little sense to me. I am glad now that I had no information about the chakras when I began to detect them, because the literature is confusing and, I have found, inaccurate, and the sources contradict one another. I suspect that several thousand years ago one or more clairvoyants mapped the fields and the information was then passed down for generations from teacher to disciple, most of whom were not clairvoyant at all. The picture I have of this transmission suggests the parlor game of Telephone, in which the first person whispers a message to the second, the second to the third and so on around a circle of people in the room until, at the end, the final message resembles the original only vaguely, if at all. The chakra information, similarly distorted, became symbolic rather than literal. Even today in India, many scholars consider the chakras to be only ideas representing stages of development in conscious awareness and not actually present in the physical body.

The chakra system is a real physical aspect of the body but very subtle in comparison to ordinary physical aspects. Many of the traditional drawings are in error as to placement of different chakras, especially the heart chakra. Some omit the spleen chakra or the lower-abdominal chakra, and none I have seen show the chakras of the knees, hands, feet, elbows and shoulders. After almost five years of exploring these energy fields, I have found more than forty such fields radiating from the body surface in the normal individual. The major chakras, however, are the ones I have described and are the ones with which I work.

After my initial three months of mapping the body's energy fields, and with the discovery that I was dealing with the ancient system of chakras, the Inner Teacher instructed me to study the disease fields of the body. I devoted the next three months to this exploration.

I discovered that I could detect disease fields by their radiation of energy only when they were in areas not in or near the major chakra areas. Cancer turned out to be the easiest kind of disease process to detect, because its field is intense and usually extends farther from the body surface than do the fields from the chakras. One can feel at a distance not only the cancer but also its metastases, if they are large enough. While benign breast lumps radiate very little or no energy, I find that highly malignant masses in the breasts are intense and to me feel hot. On the other hand, I still cannot tell the difference between an inflamed breast mass and a cancerous breast mass. Infection and cancer feel the same to me. Hepatitis radiates from a specific area over the liver, gallbladder disease from an area just below the liver. Kidney disease projects a field to the rear over the abnormal kidney. Heart disease radiates a field from the left front of the chest over the major portion of the actual heart area. Appendicitis radiates from the area where the appendix is situated.

In considering the radiation of energy from pathological tissue, there are a few general principles:

1. The abnormal fields radiate from the area where the

organ is located or the disease process is centered. I cannot detect *diffuse* disease process — such as multiple sclerosis, lupus erythematosus or leukemia — unless the disease involves and inflames a specific organ.

2. The detection of the energy field in my hands does not tell me what is wrong — only that something is wrong in that area.

3. I cannot tell from a single scan whether the process is acute or subsiding. Repeated scans are necessary to see which way the disease is going.

4. I cannot distinguish between cancer and the various forms of acute inflammation.

5. If an individual's field scan is normal, the likelihood of any major focal disease process in that body is small, unless, of course, a small focus of cancer is just beginning. In this regard I have been wrong only when the disease field was in the same location as a major chakra, e.g., a bladder tumor near the lower-abdominal chakra or cancer that has developed in a previously irradiated area of the body.

I do believe that with greater sensitivity, greater diagnostic precision is possible from simple body scans. For most people trained in science, the basic fact that disease can be detected at a distance from the body is mind-boggling enough.

Although the energy fields feel to me like heat or warmth, the radiation from these areas is not heat. They do not show up at all with thermography, in which differentials of heat radiating from the body surface are recorded photographically. In addition, this energy passes through materials that would ordinarily insulate any heat radiation, such as four-inch thick styrofoam. In fact, it passes through anything I have placed over the chakra areas, including wood, half-inch steel plates and foam rubber. (I have not yet tested with lead.) Because the energy apparently passes through anything, it is not necessary for the patient to undress to be scanned for the body fields.

Whatever the energy is, it is capable of stimulating the

sensory receptors located in the hands, forearms and other sensitive areas, such as the cheeks of the face. In me, the heat receptors are stimulated by this energy, but in other people, the cold receptors are stimulated, or the vibratory sensors, the pressure sensors or the light-touch receptors. Of more than five hundred people I have trained to sense the energy fields of the body, most feel the energy as a sensation of heat or tingling. A very few can pick up the fields only with the cheek area of their faces either as a warmth or as prickling. After completing a workshop on body-energy fields, more than 99 percent of the participants are able to sense the fields in one way or another.

Besides the failure of thermography to detect these energy fields, two other phenomena clearly prove that the fields have nothing to do with heat emanation from the body. The first is that I detected an intense field of abnormal energy, which felt like heat to my hand at a distance from the body surface, in a woman admitted to the emergency ward of the USC/L.A. County Hospital with a complete closure of the main artery of her right. leg. To the actual, physical touch, the leg felt very cold, but the field of energy radiating from it I felt as intensely hot. The second phenomenon is that the energy fields remain after death. Even after a cadaver is refrigerated for twenty-four hours, the fields are still present (though they are weaker), and they still feel like heat. I have verified this phenomenon by checking the fields of a cadaver every twelve hours for as long as three days after death. My data is too limited to draw any conclusions as to what happens to the energy fields over longer periods, but I suspect that they last as long as the body retains its physical configuration. The fields certainly remain after death; and I conclude, therefore, that they do not depend upon a viable nervous system nor upon the circulation of blood and that the energy is not of a kind currently known to science.

My interest in studying the human energy fields after death led to my first psychiatric interview. I had decided, logically enough, that the best way to determine whether the human energy fields persisted for a really long time after death was to examine some Egyptian mummies. After the Cairo Museum, the British Museum is probably the world's best repository of mummies, and so, when I was in England, I went there to scan the mummies on display.

There were a great many people milling about in that part of the building, but, undaunted, I went to work, starting with a mummy that seemed quite close to its glass enclosure. With my eyes closed, totally oblivious to my surroundings, I began to pass my hand over the surface of the glass case. What I felt confused me, for there were pectoral plates embedded with semiprecious stones on the chest area and similar plates over the abdominal incisions through which the internal organs had been removed. To make matters worse, the warmth of my own hands was reflected back to me from the glass. So, although I think I felt the chakra fields of the head and knees, I am not really sure.

When I opened my eyes to see where I was in relationship to the mummy, I saw at least twenty-five people gathered around, quietly observing me. Fortunately, the British public are polite to eccentrics. Unfortunately, the museum guard was one of the observers. I explained to him that the reflection of the ceiling lights on the glass cage interfered with my view of the mummy and I was using my hand to block the reflection and get a clearer view. From his angle, he had not been able to see that my eyes were actually closed, and he seemed to accept my explanation with only a little reluctance.

Thinking that the museum probably had many more mummies, some of them probably not protected by glass, I asked to see the head of the Egyptian antiquities department. The guard must have forewarned the official with whom I spoke, because he, without any gentle, considerate lead-in, abruptly launched the psychiatric interview. Had I been a British eccentric things would probably have gone better for me. Instead, my answers must have seemed even odder than the behavior the guard had reported. If you have traveled for long periods, you know how easy it is to know neither the day of the week nor the date — and those, of course, were two of the many questions the official asked in trying to determine my sanity. As for the names of the prime minister and the name of the queen's husband, I was a total failure. Worst of all, I could not remember who was the vice-president of the United States. To make a long story very short, I was not allowed to examine any more mummies at the British Museum.

Later I tried again in the Cairo Museum. There was a whole room full of mummies; but again, they were all in glass cases, and I got no better indication of the presence or absence of energy fields after so many years. This time, I was at least spared another psychiatric interview. A number of very curious people watched me, but here there were no guards inside the mummy room.

I believe the energy fields reflect and influence the structure of the body and its organization into organ systems. I also suspect that the chakra system is a mechanism that interrelates the gross physical body and the subtle or etheric bodies. I further believe that the chakra system, the physical body and the etheric body are in some sort of relationship with the meridians of the acupuncture system. The energy that emanates from the chakras and the energy that flows through the acupuncture meridian system are one and the same thing; the energy is either qualified by the chakra system or somehow refined by an individual chakra. I believe there is but one basic energy operating in these interrelated systems and that the chakra system modulates and transduces that basic energy. The body splays this one primary energy into its component frequencies just as the prism splays light.

This basic energy has various names: chi; vital force; nervous energy (the term the Soviet scientists use); bioenergy (the term of some American researchers); biomagnetic energy, bioelectromagnetic energy and bioplasmic energy (used by other researchers); prana (used by yogis); and Life Force (in certain metaphysical texts).

What really astounds me is that although these fields of energy have certainly been present since matter was created and life forms manifested, they still are not known to the vast majority of human beings. For that matter, it is hard for me to understand how I could have taken ten years, studying the physical body and performing so many physical examinations, before I became aware of the energy fields. At present I feel them so easily that I can't imagine why I didn't feel them before. My guess is that what held me back was that I simply didn't conceive of looking or feeling for something beyond the surface of the body. Once this idea entered my consciousness — when I thought of the possibility of feeling the warmth of the liver at a slight distance — it all began to flow. I entered a whole new world of form, matter and energy.

The study of the relationship between objects and life forms, in the physical space between them, will be a focus of science in the near future. We will discover that space is not empty but has structure and function not readily perceptible to the ordinary human awareness.

To summarize the discussion of energy fields thus far: (1) they are present in, and emanate from, the body; (2) they can be detected through several different sensory systems of the body; (3) in addition to the normal fields, there are abnormal fields that reflect disease or trauma states in the body; (4) the diagnostic potential of the abnormal energy fields depends in part upon the sensitivity of the observer; and (5) the energy fields are interrelated with the physical and etheric bodies.

With these general principles as background, I can now make a few more specific generalizations about the fields:

• People who have weak energy fields in the lower parts of their bodies, especially in the knees and feet, tend to be flighty or "spacey." Relatively ungrounded, they are disconnected to varying degrees from the outer reality system. Most of their energy is located in the upper portions of the body.

• People who have strong energy radiating from the neck area tend to be not only very sensitive to energy transfer (which I will discuss shortly) but also gifted psychically and artistically.

- Persons with strong energy radiating from the solar plexus tend to be emotional and power-driven.
- Persons with strong forehead energies tend to be mental types.
- Strong energy flow from the lower abdomen seems to indicate a sexually active individual.

I consider all these points to be in the exploratory stages of development. The correlations are not to be taken as absolute. They are my impressions now and may change as I expand my knowledge of the energy fields. There are some additional correlations related to the other chakras, but I do not consider them clearcut enough to make any statement about them.

Before I discuss the transfer of energy from one individual to another, I want to describe the classic designations of the chakra areas in case you want to correlate what I am discussing with yoga or metaphysical texts. The literature in both areas is confusing, and teachers vary in locating and numbering the chakras. Because the Sanskrit terminology is cumbersome to us, I am using the English names. (See Figs. 7.1–7.5)

0. Transpersonal point, a small ball of energy 12 to 24 inches above the center of the top of the head, not designated in most texts
1. Crown center, an area 2 to 3 inches in diameter around the center of the top of the head, the seventh level or chakra
2. Brow or forehead center, an area 1½ to 2 inches in diameter around the center of the forehead, just above the line of the eyebrows, the sixth level or chakra
3. Throat center, an area 1½ to 3 inches in diameter just above the junction of the collarbones, the fifth level or chakra
4. Upper midchest center, an area 1 to 2 inches in diameter around the junction of the manubrium and the sternum, not designated in any texts
5. Heart center, an area 1½ to 4 inches in diameter cen-

tered about 1 inch above the place where the ribs come together on the lower front part of the chest, the fourth level or chakra

6. Solar-plexus center, an area 1½ to 4 inches in diameter centered in the pit of the stomach approximately 2 inches below where the ribs come together, the third level or chakra

7. Splenic center, an area 2 to 4 inches in diameter centered over the splenic area at the edge of the lower left ribs, not usually designated with a number and often not designated at all in texts

8. Sexual center, an area 2 to 4 inches in diameter centered in the lower abdomen above the pubic bone but below the navel, the second level or chakra

9. Root center, an area 1 to 3 inches in diameter centered in the perineum, the first level or chakra

10. Hip centers, 1 to 1½ inches in diameter centered anteriorly over both hip joints, not usually designated in texts

11. Knee centers, variable in diameter and location over both knees, not designated in any texts

12. Foot centers, several in each foot, not designated in any texts

13. Shoulder centers, an area 1 to 2 inches in diameter centered over the tips of the shoulders, not designated in any texts

14. Elbow centers, over the elbows, not designated in texts

15. Hand centers, several in the fingers and the palms, not usually designated in texts

In addition to these areas where energy fields are relatively strong, there are subtler areas of radiation — from the nipple areas of women and much more subtle areas from the male breast area; from the umbilicus; from the abdomen just below the umbilicus (called the Cath center and Hara center in some books, may be very strong); from the head above the brow

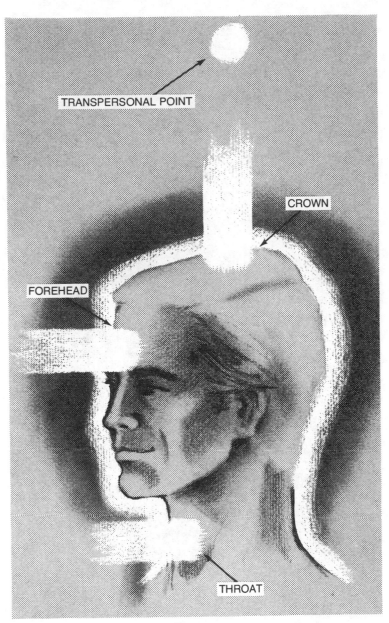

Fig. 7.1
The Major Head Chakras and Their Energy Radiations

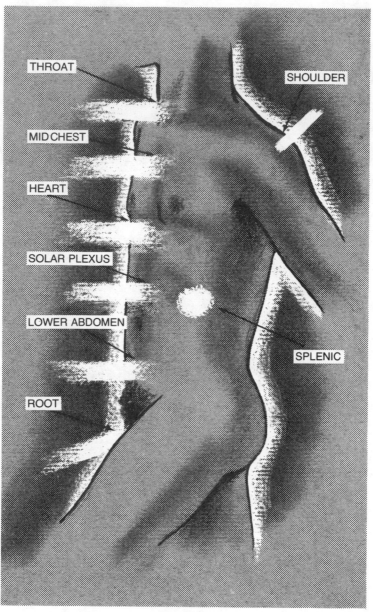

Fig. 7.2
The Major Anterior Chakras of the Trunk

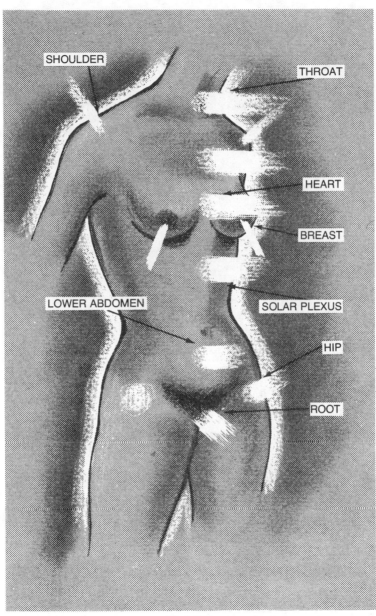

Fig. 7.3
The Major Anterior Chakras of the Trunk

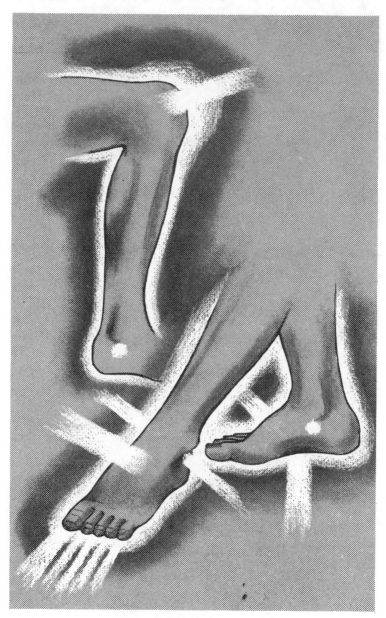

Fig. 7.4
The Major Knee and Foot Chakras

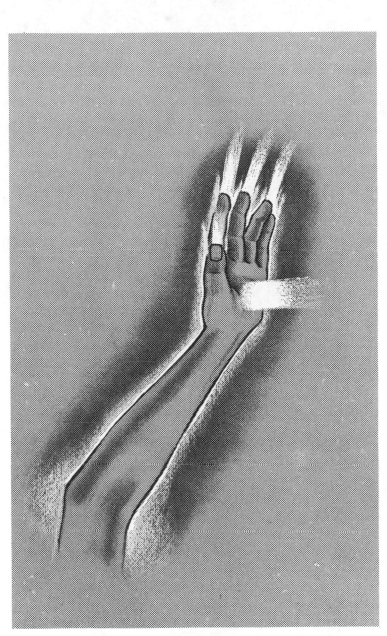

Fig. 7.5
The Hand Chakra Fields

chakra but below the crown chakra; and from the occiput area, on the back of the head above the neck or base of the skull but below the crown chakra. There are others, such as the wrist centers, the ankle centers and other centers on the face, but the numbered ones — which hips, knees, shoulders, elbows, hands and feet raise into the twenties — are the most easily located. Note that most of the secondary chakras are over joints.

Transferring energy to another person at a distance from the body is the most exciting and gratifying part of body-energy work, but it is also the most dangerous, not only to the person receiving the energy but also to the person who is transferring it. (I also want to qualify my use of the word *transfer* because I am unsure whether energy actually passes through space from one individual to another, or whether it is a process of induction or even a kind of resonance.) My own skill in this area was developed by working with extremely sensitive people who could give me feedback on what they felt as the energy went into their bodies. In the receiver, the energy can destroy or derange as easily as it can heal and harmonize. In the sender, the process of transferring energy can either deplete or overenergize the body, with bad effects either way.

Do not attempt to transfer energy to another person until you have studied thoroughly the section on techniques.

In another dialogue with the Inner Teacher, six months after the creative flash to feel for energy emanation from the body, I received the instruction to begin to share with patients the energy that flowed through my own body, directing it through my hands and working at a distance from the body, using the chakras as channels or conduits into their bodies.

During the process of scanning other bodies, or even my own, I noticed that my hands would "turn on." They would become "charged" and feel radiant. Some patients had already commented on feeling something coming from my hands as I checked their fields, but until the Inner Teacher suggested it, I had not thought of actually giving them energy. "Make all the chakra areas feel balanced and of the same intensity," the Inner

Teacher instructed me. "Go into a light meditative state and allow your intuition to tell you what to do."

I decided to begin exploring this phase with a hospitalized patient who was interested in the body-field work. After I scanned her field and noted the variations of intensity among her different chakras, I changed my state of consciousness, picked a weak chakra area and imaged energy flowing to her through my hands. Much to my amazement, and to hers, she reported a strong feeling, almost like an electric current, flowing into and through her body from the area where I was working. The chakra, when I checked it again, was greatly intensified. If I didn't *will* the energy to flow from my hands but simply imaged it and *allowed* it to flow, the energy seemed to stop flowing when the correct intensity was reached.

When I finished, I felt energized and sensed a high state of well-beingness and inspiration. My own heart chakra was highly charged with energy and seemed to be the source from which the energy flowed into my hands and on to the patient. I felt the same alteration of my Beingness as I had felt when I was bathed by the radiance of Eunice, when she was in a state of Unconditional Love.

My patient reported the sensation of having been placed in an altered state of consciousness, as if she were levitating, floating several feet above her body. She described the energy as "loving and healing." She had not previously experienced the sensation of levitation, but it later turned out to be a fairly common experience when I balanced chakras in other patients.

As I continued to balance people's chakras over the next month, I was truly awed by the individual differences in effect. Some reported "blisslike" states, some profound relaxation, some dreamlike states in vivid color, some intense heat pouring through their bodies, some a loss of consciousness. A few experienced nothing at all, although I clearly felt the flow of energy leaving my body. And even though they felt no sensation, their chakra fields were altered and balanced by the transfer. I could feel the difference when I rescanned them.

There was very little in any literature on using the chakra-balancing energy for the alteration of disease fields, but between my office practice and my hospital cases, there were ten instances where I felt that balancing the chakras by itself — that is, without any particular intention of altering the disease field — had in fact made a difference in the disease process. I was not interested, really, in proving that point, or any other. I simply wanted to continue to explore the possibilities of energy work. Keep in mind that I did not know what the energy that radiated from the chakras was, nor did I know what the energy that seemed to flow from my hands was. I did not know how the energy could produce altered states of consciousness in myself or in the patient, much less in both. To summarize the status of my work at that time, I really did not know what I was doing.

I decided for two reasons to use energy-field work with cancer patients. The first was that medicine could do only so much for most cancer patients. Much treatment was only palliative. While patients and their families might have felt real hope for cure, there was very little of it in the consciousness of the physicians who were treating them. If energy work was helpful in such a desperate situation, it could not be criticized, however radical or unconventional. The patients, most of them, had nothing to lose.

The second reason for concentrating on cancer was that cancer's field of energy is easily detected, so that the scanning procedure is a simple matter. As far as I could explain it to them, the patients were fully informed as to what I was doing, and no conventional therapy was withdrawn: energy therapy did not replace any orthodox approach. Because conventional treatment was continued and because I combined Command Therapy with the energy-field work, it was almost impossible to determine which technique was causing what effect; but that question didn't bother me. I was interested solely in bringing to patients whatever could help them.

At that time I had only begun the deep psychological probe into the consciousness of the cancer patient, but I already saw a clear general trend. Most of them had experienced traumatic emotional events within two years before the onset of their disease — loss of a job, loss of a loved one, children leaving home, moving away from a lifelong environment and the like. Brief, highly emotional events were not as important in the cancer background as were deep, prolonged, stressful traumas. Besides the changes that the patients wanted in their disease processes, they all desired major changes in their lives.

That year of exploration, 1973–74, altered my entire approach to health and disease. Occasionally the truly miraculous occurred; in a few cases, I could actually feel a tumor mass simply melting under my hands. In the majority of cases, the tumor seemed to stabilize or show little change; while there was no great remission, at least the cancer's growth was arrested. In many patients, unfortunately, nothing seemed to stop the disease process. But all the patients, even the clearly terminal ones, reported that they were less depressed, all had less fear of death and a number could finally realize that death was just what they wanted. Those people were relieved that they could at last, without guilt, express this feeling to someone.

Early on in the process of working so deeply with dying patients, I realized that my own attitudes about death and my own fears were precipitating a countertransference reaction in me. That is, I was taking on some of the negative feelings of my patients. I placed myself in the hands of a woman therapist, and she not only gave me insight into the countertransference phenomenon, but initiated a deep probe into the psychological patterns that worked against me in my relationships with others.

I discovered that my ability to share my Beingness with others who were sick depended critically upon the state of my own consciousness and sense of well-being. After this insight, I taught myself to move to an inspired state of awareness at will, especially when working with patients. It was a disciplined action. When I worked with body energies, my state of consciousness was always the same, a state of Unconditional Love and inspiration.

I also learned that the relationship between the physician or healer and the patient is a two-way exchange. Patients were as responsible for accepting and responding to the therapeutic agents and energy work as I was for delivering the energy and other therapeutic modalities to their bodies for healing. In whatever form of treatment, the patient is not simply passive. He or she must clear the psychological areas that were factors in precipitating the disease and are factors in perpetuating it. The pattern configurating the factors that allow disease to manifest in the body is not in the outer awareness of the patient. It is deeply buried. Patients can yell from the rooftops that they want to get well, or that they are innocent of the events that are transpiring in them, but I know differently. People are never innocent of what happens to them.

The memory in the subconscious and unconscious areas of any human being transcends, almost beyond comprehension, the memory of this particular brief span of awareness called a lifetime. To the vaster memory, specifics are unimportant. Patterns alone are what matter. We are all interwoven into one another's patterns, we have been for generations and we will be for generations in the future. When we learn to heal and to harmonize our relationships both internally and externally, it becomes possible to transform and transcend the human plane.

When you can forgive both another and yourself, the pattern is broken, and you move from the law of karma (action and reaction) into the law of grace (resolution) — that effulgent state that transmutes and heals. Intrinsic to Unconditional Love — the fourth state of awareness, the heart-chakra state of consciousness — is forgiveness. No amount of rationalizing, no matter what the extent, can really forgive. In unified consciousness there are no deceptions. We see our underlying motivations and so can allow Love to marshal the healing powers that are ours to wield. The outer conditioned mind alone cannot do it. It must be connected with what can only be called the spiritual aspect; then the honesty cards must be drawn to see clearly whether the unconscious and subconscious balance of forces is for transformation through death or through the life process. (These aspects will be discussed further in Chapter Nine.)

Energy transfer can also affect pain in the body. Oddly, it wasn't until January 1976 that I realized that the energy flowing from my hands could relieve any pain at all. It does not matter whether the pain is stress-induced, as with muscular aches or the pain and headaches caused by tension or produced by some organic process, from cancer to broken bones and torn ligaments to the pain of surgery. Usually the pain can be totally relieved within a few minutes. In some cases the relief is permanent, but more often it lasts from several hours to several days. I have worked with an orthopedic surgeon on a skiing-accident patient, setting a fracture of both bones of a lower leg without using any drugs to kill the pain. In addition, muscular relaxation allowed the fracture to be set easily and with little discomfort to the patient.

It is easy to teach others how to transfer this pain-relieving energy, but, ultimately, we will discover how to capture this energy spectrum — perhaps through some device similar to and as simple as a tape recorder — and then to amplify it and direct it to areas of chronic or acute pain, so that we will have total control of pain without narcotics or even analgesics. The human instrument can do it now, but mechanical instruments will be developed in the future to do the same thing.

There are several wondrous aspects of the pain relief achieved with this technique, producing normal sensation in and around the previously painful areas. In cases of repeated use, unlike narcotics, it does not seem to require more energy and last for shorter time periods; there is no habituation to it. And it leaves the mind of the patient totally clear.

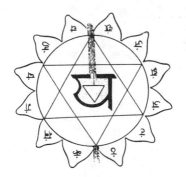

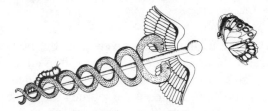

Meditation, Breath Control, the Spiral Meditation, Quickening, Protection and Shielding

*"Ponderability is inversely
proportional to substantiality."*
— Franklin Merrell-Wolff

Because I have already mentioned meditation several times, you may wonder why it has taken me so long to get to a chapter of specific discussion and instruction on the subject. I hope that as you read this chapter you will realize that the previous chapters gave information necessary to understand and to use this one.

If, on the other hand, you got to this chapter by looking at the table of contents or the index and turning to the subject that interested you most, I advise you to start at the beginning of the book and read up to this point if you want to understand it and get the most value from it.

Meditation is the empowering experience. In the stead of the narrow path of the outer-mind journey, with its many endless circles and its culs-de-sac, meditation is the journey to the

179

everywhere of the entire universe, to the nowhere of the infinitesimal point at the center of the individual consciousness, and it joins the everywhere and the nowhere demonstrating they both are one. Meditation is the journey into the essence of all, a spiral ever expanding into dimensions and experiences of awareness beyond the self, beyond thought forms, beyond time, beyond fear, beyond death, sometimes exploding into the superbrilliant light of Ascension, unshackling through Resurrection, to where Self abides.

In meditation, the pinhole of outer awareness begins to merge into the small aperture of self, which then begins to emerge through the wider lens of the collective, on through a great circle that is only a pore of the Cosmic, and goes on into the Light.

To experience at will the naturally induced states of higher consciousness, to shift from the self to Self by nothing more than the lowering of the eyelids, to experience the melting of one solid definition into the soft, amorphous, undefined, to begin to claim one's inheritance as a conscious universal entity — all can be accomplished through the art of meditation. I call it an art, because it is not a skill, as so many people believe. It is not available at all to people who know only the outer conditioned aspect of the mind or who fear their own mortality. Meditation is Divinity's playground.

Teachers throughout the ages have warned the aspirant that, as empowering by meditation commences, the inner eye must be kept on the golden thread that guides the awareness into awakening, on through enlightenments and finally to illumination. Attachment to any preliminary level of awareness along the way initiates a process to return toward the level of the outer mind. Detachment is a ticket Home.

As a beginning experience in meditation, as two or more levels of awareness begin to play off one another, the mind erects paradoxes difficult to believe, impossible to describe. Each aspect of the paradox is comprehensible only from its own level of perception so that the two (or more) sides can never meet; but an inner necessity drives one deeper to more expanded

states. And there, on a still deeper level, a single insight resolves the dichotomy.

Other experiences of meditation are:
• What is madness to one soul is bliss to another
• One's various component aspects all at once in dialogue
with one another
• Guides, teachers, angels and demons
• The comprehension of poetry or poetic language attempting to describe sublime or mystical states — a language that is almost, if not downright, irrational to the
linear mind
• Chatter, seemingly endless chatter, and then the contrast of silence into Silence

Meditation is, finally, an infinite experience for the awareness
to explore.

There are as many different ways to meditate as there are
meditators. One excellent book on the more classical approaches is *The Varieties of the Meditative Experience* by
Daniel Goleman. I recommend it for its conciseness but not
necessarily for its inclusiveness. There are many, many books
on the subject — so many in fact, that I prefer simply to discuss
my own appraoch first with a general description, then with
step-by-step directions.

You have an innate ability to meditate. It is not something
you have to learn how to do. You do have to allow time for the
experience, but, in essence, you do not have to structure the act
itself.

I did not meditate until January 1972, when Eunice, in one
of her public classes, suggested that we begin by going into
meditation for twenty-five minutes. There were a hundred
people there, and the ninety-nine others all seemed to know
what to do.

"Begin your relaxation process with breath control,"
Eunice instructed us.

"What on earth is breath control?" I asked myself. I

suspected, with apprehension, that I was probably the only one in the entire audience who had never meditated before.

Eunice told us to take our shoes off, sit straight in our chairs, with both feet on the floor, our hands relaxed, palms up on our thighs and our eyes closed and to b-r-e-a-t-h-e. "In through the nose slowly," said Eunice. Everyone took in a slow deep breath through the nose. "That's it. A little deeper. Expand the chest fully. Feel the prana [energy] enter your lungs. Now hold your breath."

I was obviously doing it wrong. I had reached the full expansion of my lungs long before anybody else, and I was already feeling the need to exhale and take in another breath.

"Now hold the breath for a slow count of seven," Eunice said gently.

"I'm going to faint!" I thought. I tried to relax into her *very* slow count of seven.

"Feel the energy flood your body," Eunice was saying in between counts four and five.

"What energy?" I was thinking. "All my energy has been used up!"

"You are all doing so well," Eunice serenely continued. "That's it. Six. Seven. Now slowly exhale through the mouth, with the tongue touching the roof of the mouth. Be sure there is a quiet hissing sound as you slowly exhale."

The sound I produced was more like a high-powered exhaust fan, but by then I didn't care. All I could think about was how to empty my lungs fast enough to be able to get more air in. "Slowly now," Eunice directed. "Don't exhale too rapidly. Keep your awareness on the energy that is now entering every cell of your body."

"If I don't get some air quickly, somebody is going to have to resuscitate me!" I screamed silently to myself. "This is ridiculous. If I can breathe very quietly, without anybody else knowing, maybe I can catch my breath." So I began to breathe as quietly as possible, but as rapidly as possible, without making too much of a sound.

I was sneaking in two breaths for every one that the rest of the class was taking. "You are not doing it right," Eunice said lovingly. She did not mention my name, but I could feel her voice aimed directly at me. How could she possibly know? I opened my eyes to see that she was indeed looking at me. I smiled.

"Close your eyes, Brugh, and see if you can catch up with the group." She said it so smoothly that she never for a second lost track of the group or missed a single count. Slowly, I took in a deep breath and felt an energy surge into my lungs. Holding my breath for a count of seven was suddenly easy. I could concentrate my attention on the energy that seemed to be flooding my body as I slowly exhaled, and now I, too, could make the appropriate soft hissing sound. It was a wonderful sensation, completely achieved by the time she finished with the breathing exercise and told us to breathe naturally and quietly and to let our awareness gently relax into a quiet, clear pool of warm water.

I don't remember anything after that. I was off into my first exploration of expanded awareness, totally blanked out. I next remember Eunice saying, "Come out now...That's it...Slowly feel yourself enter your body...Begin to move your hands, arms and legs...That's it...Fine...Is everyone back? Some of you are not coming out...Twenty-five minutes is enough in the beginning stages."

"Twenty-five minutes!" I thought. It seemed like two or three minutes. My outer mind was confused. Wherever I had gone, it gave the impression of being deep, serene and nourishing. My outer mind thought that I had probably fallen asleep, but my deeper intuition told me differently. I had entered a state of consciousness beyond the outer awareness. I had to trust that what had happened was beneficial.

Eunice told me after class that she had hardly been able to keep from laughing as she watched my energy field at the beginning of the meditation. She said, in fact, that she had directed some energy to me to allow me to relax into the exercise. I was convinced because I knew that as soon as she had looked at me something had happened. The sense of being out of breath had suddenly been dissipated.

When I told her that I had blanked out, she seemed pleased.

"Oh, that's wonderful, Brugh. One of the highest forms of meditation is loss of awareness." This reassuring explanation did not satisfy my outer mind. It was too busy being incensed that it had not been able to participate, but my body did feel unusually relaxed and vital, and my mind — my whole mind — experienced clarity and a sense of harmony.

There are some significant points about this first meditation:

First and most important, I trusted Eunice more than any other living person. Her presence ignited me. I don't think I could have let go of the control of my outer mind without this trust.

When we all entered into the quiet breathing part of the exercise, I was not aware of body boundaries. I felt expanded and fluid. I was floating in that warm, clear pool of water, unaware that I was in a room with many other people.

Somehow my consciousness fused into the group field. Individuality had disappeared — and I didn't care.

And, finally, Eunice radiated confidence and mastery. Her words at the beginning of the experience dispelled my anxiety.

I have realized since then that a group meditative field consistently induces a meditative state in anyone sitting in or near the group, if the person will allow his or her awareness to relax. So, if you wish to experience meditation quickly and easily, find an experienced meditation group and join it. Just sitting next to even one person who is meditating can be enough.

Eunice taught that the state of Unconditional Love, once it was experienced, could be utilized as the center post of awareness to allow the exploration of any state of consciousness in meditation. As long as one was encapsulated in Love, nothing experienced in meditation could be detrimental. My own experience has proved this generalization to be true. One can get into some really frightening states — and other states, where one holds on to other emotions — but the impersonal state of Love allows their exploration without reaction.

Each morning in a two-week Conference, an hour for meditation is set aside between 6:00 and 7:00 A.M. People who want this experience are invited to meditate in the seminar room, a large space, the floor double-padded and carpeted, with huge pillows on which to sit. The hour is one of complete silence on the entire ranch, so that people who find meditation difficult with conversation or noisy activity can enjoy the quiet. It is not mandatory that everyone meditate in the more formal sense at that hour or any other. I have found that many people enter meditative states while walking or while doing T'ai Chi, swimming or jogging. Many who have never meditated before, do find the energy of the seminar room conducive to the experience.

My personal preference is to quiet myself and — without forging a pathway into some preconceived idea about what should be experienced in meditation — to allow my awareness to be guided into the expanded states by that portion of my consciousness that really knows. Most important, I do not try to discriminate whether I am in a meditative or a contemplative state of awareness, or whether anything is happening. I trust that the higher aspects of my Beingness, as they direct the experience, will bring to my awareness what is necessary for my development into the highest potential for this lifetime. I do not try to define what that potential is, nor am I concerned that my potential in this lifetime may not be total illumination. In meditation, I do not feel fulfilled; I feel more that I am forever in a continuing, never completed, process of being fulfilled.

Fundamentally, the experience of meditation teaches the outer awareness how to shift its perspectives both horizontally and vertically. Within one (vertical) level of awareness, many different (horizontal) perspectives are available. One doesn't, however, have to try out all the horizontal perspectives in that level; a few can suffice. The shift to a higher (vertical) level gives new dimensional perspectives (that is, a new and different set of horizontal perspectives) with an overview vaster than that available on the lower, less expanded level. As a rule, attachment to one level leads to horizontal explorations, while detachment activates the vertical explorations.

Meditation is a tool of the consciousness, not an end in

itself. Do the kind of meditation that intuitively feels right to do, whether it is formal posturing or a quiet nature walk. As has been documented time and time again, cosmic awareness happens whether you meditate or not. You don't make it happen; it happens to you. All you really have to do is get out of the way and stop blocking your own unfolding development.

A few other suggestions may be helpful. Meditating while lying in bed in the morning is generally (but not always) ineffective. For most people, the horizontal position is too strongly associated with sleep and the hypnagogic borderline of sleep, which are not meditative states. Some research studies seem to indicate that the sitting position — whether cross-legged, in the East Indian lotus position or even in a chair — increases the alertness of consciousness for meditation.

If the mind persists in chattering away, interfering with meditation, I recommend creating for the chatter inside a huge auditorium filled with people. Don't be stingy about the size of the auditorium or the number of people you create. Then just tell the chatterer to talk to all those people and to keep them entertained while you go ahead with your meditation. All the chatterer wants is an audience; so by splitting your consciousness into a portion that listens and the vaster portion that doesn't have to listen, the problem can often be overcome. This method works far better than trying to kill the chatterer — an act that requires a great deal more energy than it takes to create the large auditorium packed with people. The less importance you give to the mind chatterer, the greater the opportunity of overcoming this common disruption of meditation.

Meditating on a full stomach is almost impossible. You will find that meditation is easier to get into, and feels much more expanded, on an empty stomach. For most people the early morning hours are the most conducive to deep meditative states. After a morning meditation, one's day is apt to have a feeling of greater serenity.

The meditative state not only induces profound relaxation but also clears mental and physical fatigue. As a result, meditation before bedtime reduces the need for sleep. In fact, the hyperaware state that follows meditation sometimes makes it difficult to fall asleep. If you wish to meditate more often than just in the morning, I suggest you avoid evening sessions. Try late afternoon periods instead.

How much time you spend in meditation is up to you. At first, allow an hour of quiet time. If you find that your meditation is over in ten minutes, don't just sit for the rest of the hour with your mind whirling on the day's activities; get up and start your day. Some days your meditation will sweep you into a timeless state where the hour will seem like minutes.

I recommend a beginning meditation by feeling into what the experience of Unconditional Love would be like if one were to enter this state of awareness. Other experiences will begin to appear as the technique develops. Gandhi is supposed to have said that five minutes in meditation, contemplating Unconditional Love, would do more for the world than filling starving people's rice bowls. My outer, limited material mind might say, "Ridiculous!" to Gandhi's statement, but my inner vision knows the power of Love. It agrees with Gandhi.

During a personal counseling session with Eunice, I felt a most overwhelming inpouring of Love. Eunice paused, then said, "Brugh, if you only knew how many people over many, many lifetimes have sent Unconditional Love to you, knowing that at some time your Beingness would open to that Love! What you are feeling is all of their Love flooding your awareness. It is happening now because you have, in this moment, opened to it. Love sent to another soul surrounds that soul, awaiting the time when the outer mind of that individual opens the door. No one can open the door for another."

Tears poured from my eyes. I knew she spoke the truth. I was swept into a state of bliss beyond words. Love cannot be overemphasized either in meditation or in the outer experience of Life.

In general, there are two broad, mutually exclusive approaches to meditation. In the first, one excludes or blocks out from the awareness any outer sound or activity. One simply tunes out everything. This technique requires a quiet space. The second approach is inclusive, and utilizes all sound and action to heighten the meditative state. It is used in the practice of Zen meditation. I prefer this second approach because I find that with it I can take any energy — such as the sound of conversation, music or a telephone ringing — and transmute it into a catapult to take me into deeper states of awareness. This approach also enables me to meditate anywhere and at any time.

Breath control in itself is a really amazing experience. If one does it properly, the lightness one feels is not caused by hyperventilation. Instead, something else indefinable happens. I know from my own experience that the body-energy fields are modified by controlled breathing and that modulation of the breath can modulate the flow of energy from the hands. As you go on, you will probably have this experience yourself. Experiment with it.

My initial meditation with Eunice was as I described it. Step-by-step directions may help you to use it directly, too. You are going to perform a series of ten controlled breaths. Seated in a chair or on the floor in any of the ways described, with your shoes off and your eyes closed, begin to inhale slowly through your nose. When your lungs are fully expanded, hold your breath without tension while you slowly count to seven, and then slowly exhale through your mouth, with your tongue touching the front of the roof of the mouth so that you make a slight hissing noise. Exhale slowly and completely, and then start the cycle over again. Repeat it for a total of ten times. This technique is a wonderful way to attune and prepare the awareness for any meditation.

Breath control can be a meditation in itself if it is carried out for a period of time, but I prefer to use it as a beginning, a way to relax into whatever form of meditation I may choose at a given moment. After the cycle of ten breaths, one might, for example, begin the contemplation of Unconditional Love, or one might practice the visualization technique, already discussed, of pinning numbers of a blank curtain. One could just "let go and let God" — not focusing or doing anything but sitting quietly, sensing after well-beingness — or one could begin the spiral meditation, which is to be presented later in this chapter.

Remember, however, that meditation, any meditation, is over when you begin to reenter ordinary awareness, when the expanded state feels as if it is waning. Don't try to stop the reentry. There is always another opportunity for another deepening meditation. You will find that there are times when five minutes is too long and other times when an hour isn't long enough!

In the exploration of the higher dimensions of consciousness, balance is a key concept, and balance in the hours spent in meditation is important. I very often see people trying to achieve some sort of state of enlightenment through the practice of prolonged meditation without proper guidance. What these people do not understand is that trying is not the mechanism by which higher states are achieved. They are achieved through the mechanism of *allowing*. Too much forced meditation, instead of expanding the consciousness, can fatigue the mind and body, sometimes inducing states of psychosis that are difficult to clear. There are times I consciously give myself permission not to meditate in the morning. I don't whip myself or feel guilty about it. Something inside me knows when my attention needs to be focused on matters in the outer plane. But I always set aside an hour each morning for the experience, whether I meditate or not.

Part of the meditative experience is the development of the *witness state*, and Unconditional Love is one pathway to it. In the witness state, an impersonal observer can be found within one's awareness. It simply observes, without reaction to whatever passes before the awareness. It usually cannot be achieved, or further developed, without Unconditional Love or, as you may realize, without the three admonitions heard by the clairvoyant woman on the Santa Monica beach.

As I have already said, Unconditional Love is totally unemotional and impersonal. Yet there is an inexplicable and indescribable feeling to it. The feeling is beyond a sense of integration, intimacy and inspiration; but it includes those feeling tones—in, however, a nonemotional nature.

From this witness state it is possible to go even farther, to a place where not even compassion is felt. This state is the *high indifference* that Western mystic Franklin Merrell-Wolff discusses in his books, *Pathway Through to Space* and *The Philosophy of Consciousness Without an Object*. As he says—and I am paraphrasing—the state is so inhuman that few people ever venture to develop it. Although it seems contrary to all our impulses toward feelings for others—and even ourselves—it is an essential tool to master, because high indifference brings a detail of observation and a clarity of insight unattainable by any other means.

Many people have inquired about my Inner Teacher with which I dialogue in some meditations. Although the specific aspects of my teacher don't really matter at all, it is very important to realize that one can contact or create one's own Inner Teacher. After Eunice died, I realized that no more outer teacher was possible for me, and my total intention in meditation then was to allow my consciousness to carry me into the discovery of an Inner Teacher. The basic conception and my allowing of it were all that were necessary for the experience to occur. In such matters, one's individual consciousness is capable of the most magnificent expressions. Trust it.

In this case, trust the state of awareness you begin to experience centered around the level and experiences of the heart chakra. Of the many voices inside everybody, some are the voices of people we know or voices we know to be our own chatterers inside; but there is complication, even danger, if one is not opening to the honesty of one's Beingness. When one is deceiving oneself, there are voices that are not going to be helpful. They can be dangerous, because they tell us to do all sorts of things that have nothing to do with any reality except a concocted one of our own making. Everyone exploring higher awareness passes through thought areas that may have voices associated with them. We can and must learn to ignore the negative or erroneous voices. It is a painstaking process from which no one escapes. Keeping your intention clearly on the heart area and exploration of Love will greatly simplify this developmental sequence for you.

The *spiral meditation* came to me one morning in Findhorn as I was dialoguing with the Inner Teacher on the subject of chakras. During the meditation, I received an image of a naked man standing with his arms extended out from his sides. From the area of his heart chakra, a pattern of energy began to form. It flowed to the man's left and down in a spiral pattern to his solar-plexus chakra; continued to the right and up to the mid-chest chakra; then left and down to the splenic chakra; right and down to the lower-abdomen chakra; right and up to the throat chakra; and so on in the spiral to the root chakra, the forehead chakra, then to the left elbow, left knee, right knee, right elbow; on up to the crown chakra and around on to the left hand, left foot, right foot, right hand; and finally to an area about eighteen inches above the head, the transpersonal point. (See Fig. 8.1.)

The vision was beautiful: all the major and important chakras were connected in a single spiral pattern. The Inner Teacher told me that I was to work with my own chakra system in this same sequence at the beginning of my meditations, and at the end, to reverse the flow and pattern of the spiral, working from the transpersonal point back to the heart. (See Fig. 8.2.)

It is the sole flowing geometric pattern that includes the splenic chakra. And I find it interesting that the heart contracts in a twisting spiral fashion, not like a pump, and that the basic DNA molecule is a double helix, a modification of the spiral. During fetal development, the lower extremities in humans are twisted in a partial spiral so that the knee is rotated 180 degrees in relationship to the elbow. On the grand scale, we are moving through space in a series of simultaneous spirals — and we are situated in a symmetrical spiral galaxy.

In the classical literature of metaphysics, the Egyptians, Japanese, Tibetans and Sufis all teach that the center of the body is in the abdomen, near or just below the umbilicus, and many

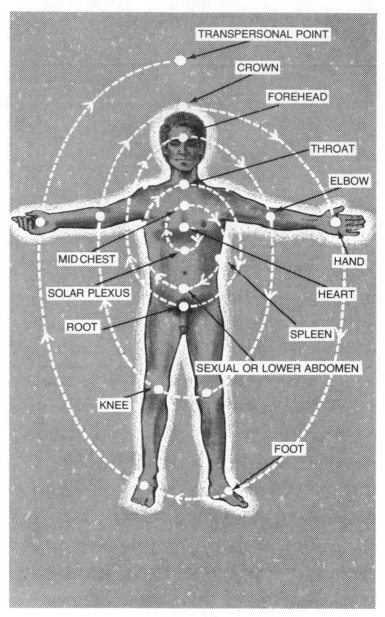

TRANSPERSONAL POINT

CROWN

FOREHEAD

THROAT

ELBOW

HAND

MID CHEST

SOLAR PLEXUS

HEART

ROOT

SPLEEN

SEXUAL OR LOWER ABDOMEN

KNEE

FOOT

Fig. 8.1
Opening Spiral Pattern

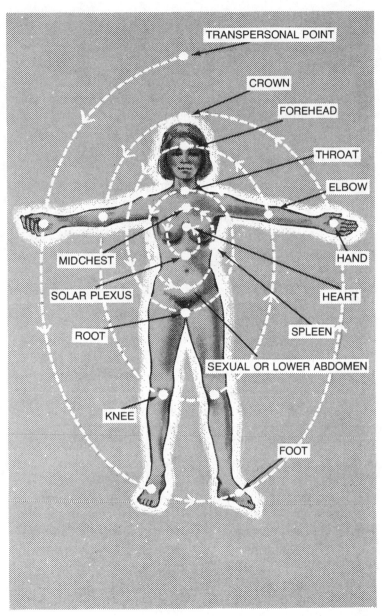

TRANSPERSONAL POINT

CROWN

FOREHEAD

THROAT

ELBOW

MIDCHEST

HAND

SOLAR PLEXUS

HEART

ROOT

SPLEEN

SEXUAL OR LOWER ABDOMEN

KNEE

FOOT

Fig. 8.2
Closing Spiral Pattern

present-day students of metaphysics believe that the ancient scriptures are still to be followed exactly as they were two thousand to twenty-five hundred years ago. My placing of the center of energy awareness at the heart center quite obviously contradicts these old teachings. I believe that the consciousness of human beings has evolved and is evolving, and that the point of focus is shifting from a point below the diaphragm to a point above the diaphragm. I see no need at this time to reestablish and reinforce what essentially was the level of development thousands of years ago. We are preparing for a transformation of consciousness that supersedes the past, moving from the more power-controlled areas, the areas of mastery of the material plane, into a blend with the higher awareness that is associated with the upper chakras. The root chakra, the sexual chakra and the solar-plexus—splenic chakras comprise the lower triangle; it is associated primarily with the physical and emotional planes. The heart, throat, forehead and crown chakras are associated with the developing spiritual awareness of humanity. The heart chakra, the fourth level, sits midway between the lower triangle and the main upper chakras. This shift of the center upward will imbue humanity with a sense of relationship, the deeper aspects of which rest on spiritual values rather than on power and control over others.

Humanity has been in a transitional state of awakening since the last century. Transitional states are always chaotic as the cadavers of old, rigid institutions begin to crumble and the new vision comes into its birthing process. Change, no matter how painful, is essential to life, and change is what we are just beginning to experience now. The statement that humanity's fulcrum has moved upward, across and past the diaphragm, may be painful to traditionalists, but so, to earlier traditionalists, was the realization that the earth is not the center of the universe. As I said previously, most of our Beingness is not centered in the physical body. The shift to the heart is a beginning reflection of this actuality, a shift to a relationship between the body and the spirit.

So, in the spiral meditation, you center your awareness in

humankind's approaching center, the heart-chakra area, leaving behind personal concerns and entering into a more universal state of consciousness. As awareness rests into the heart chakra, you sense a feeling of warmth, expansion or vibration in that area. In my experience, working with my own chakras in morning meditation, I do not leave the heart chakra until I feel that it is fully activated, guiding my awareness into Unconditional Love for all Life. With this activation, there is an almost orgasmic sensation in the area of the chakra. I then envision the beginning of the spiral energy pattern carrying the essence of the heart chakra to the solar plexus, focusing my attention on it until it is activated. I repeat this process, going to each successive chakra in the spiral and waiting until it feels activated, again with the physical sensation that is closer to bliss than to orgasm. After I have proceeded through the activation of all the chakras in the spiral pattern, I finally rest at the transpersonal point and relax totally into a meditative state. Later, when I am ready to conclude the meditation, I begin at the transpersonal point and, working through the spiral in the opposite direction, prepare each chakra for its integration into the physical plane until, reaching the heart chakra, I experience a sense of expanded appreciation for the opportunity to be alive, embodied and spiritually quickened. I rededicate my Beingness to service to humankind.

There are more advanced steps possible in the spiral meditation, but the ones I have outlined here are the basic ones I work with each morning. The natural order of the awakening of the chakras is not, as often taught, in a straight-line, stepladder pattern up from the root to the crown and back down again.

In the natural pattern as I see it, the chakras are awakened in ascending pairs. First, the second (sexual) chakra is transformed to the fifth (throat), reflecting the transformation from physical procreative activity to such aesthetic creativity as art, literature and music. The second transformation is from the third chakra (solar plexus) to the fourth (heart), reflecting the change from emphasis on power and the emotional aspects of awareness to the more collective and unconditioned states of awareness, imbued with Love. Finally, the first chakra (root) is activated, its energies ascending to the seventh (crown). There are effects on the head centers with the first two transformations; but the third, the root to the crown, represents the unbelievable energy variously called the Fire, the Serpent Fire, the Kundalini energy, the Fire of Transformation. When it is fully activated and begins to ascend through the energy pathways, connecting each of the successive chakras, the process is called the rising of the Kundalini. It sweeps the individual into cosmic states of awareness.

The Kundalini energy can also be awakened through a willed action. This uncontrolled awakening, in someone who has not prepared the higher chakras for such an intensity of energy, can be devastating, causing not only great physical pain but psychological pain as well. Gopi Krishna's book *The Kundalini: The Evolutionary Energy in Man* clearly demonstrates the consequences of awakening this last transformational energy surge in an individual who was unprepared.

It is important at this point to discriminate between *active* chakras and *awakened* chakras. Even in the most unawakened individual, all the chakras in the human being are active; but in most people, they function primarily in relation to the physical body in the physical manifest plane and, in the more subtle manifest plane, to the etheric body. These chakras are in what is called a dormant or resting state of activity. Despite the terminology, energy activity from these dormant or resting chakras is readily felt with the scanning technique. An awakened chakra is functioning at an entirely different level of activity. An awakened chakra not only feels different in scanning, it looks different to clairvoyant vision.

If some of this material sounds familiar, especially to one who has read Alice Bailey, I make no apology. Whoever and whatever my Inner Teacher is, it obviously is familiar with the concepts channeled not only by Alice Bailey but by Rudolf Steiner, Edgar Cayce and others, as well. I was amazed when in January 1977 I read Alice Bailey's book *Esoteric Healing* and found in it many concepts that I had received from the Inner Teacher and had already been teaching in my Conference work.

Several physical phenomena are associated with the focusing of the energy flow in the body. They can be inexplicable and frightening experiences. A discussion of them may give the reader some insight as to what to expect. It is important to emphasize once again the necessity of clearly setting one's intention to experience the heart chakra awareness and not to be seduced by any of the byproducts that may manifest along the way.

The Quakers are called Quakers because, when in a form of spiritual ecstacy, they quake. The Shakers are called Shakers because, in a similar state, they shake. Others call this quaking or shaking phenomenon "quickening," and it is similar to, if not the same as, the reaction that can occur in the opening process in Subud and in other forms of induction (or initiation) that produce an altered or heightened state of consciousness. Often this physical reaction appears spontaneously anywhere from several months to several years after one begins daily meditation. The muscular response is not volitional, and it stops if the state of consciousness is broken. Recently I have been hearing about more and more people—people who do not meditate and who have never heard or read about such a phenomenon—who have had this experience, especially at night in bed.

For me, the quickening began within a few weeks after I first met Eunice. I was sure that the big California earthquake had struck. I jumped out of bed and was heading for safety when I realized that nothing in the room seemed disturbed—in particular, a hanging light fixture in my room wasn't swinging. The same thing happened several nights in succession, and each time it startled me. My whole bed seemed to shake. I always checked my pulse to see whether I was having heart palpitations, and my heartbeat was always regular. Finally I had to conclude that my body was shaking or going into strange repetitive muscular contractions. When I told Eunice, she laughed and said, "Oh, that's just the beginning of the inpouring of energy in preparation for your eventual awakening." I still have similar experiences, but over time they have been modified. Now the sensation is like a very fine motor or fast vibration centered at different times in different areas of my body, primarily in the chest, neck and forehead areas.

This phenomenon must be differentiated from the ordinary muscle twitches and occasional spasms everybody feels. It is also to be differentiated from the "restless-leg" syndrome, which physicians usually diagnose in older people. Their legs simply won't stay still during the night. Quinine usually remedies this situation, but it won't influence the quickening phenomenon; I tried it.

The most spectacular experience I have had, in association with the quickening phenomenon, is what I call the superbrilliant light space.

In a morning meditation in February 1976, I had the sensation of a motor turning on in my chest area, and then I saw a momentary flash of blinding white light. In each subsequent meditation, and each night just after I went to bed, I experienced the same blindingly intense flash of light; it was far more intense than looking at the sun or at any other brilliantly lighted object I had ever seen. I began to try to hold the light in my awareness, but I could not do it. The light was just too bright. A second was more than I could stand.

The experience, sometimes skipping a few days but always of the same quality, continued until November 1976. Then, one night, I was lying in bed, just about to fall asleep, when the motor came on; but this time it was not the usual motor. This time it was like a Diesel truck. Its vibration shook not only me, but also the kingsize bed. It was first centered in my chest area, then moved into the lower abdomen, then up toward my head. On came the superbrilliant light. It was not just a flash, and it did not stop. For a moment, I was terrified. Then I heard a voice say, "What do you think you have been preparing for?" I accepted it and relaxed into the experience. It lasted for about six hours: intense, intense, intense white light and the quaking of my whole body. The next morning, I felt unusually rested and nothing appeared grossly different to my awareness; but over the next few months I recognized that my work was maturing, and my ability to see energy fields was beginning to increase. Something subtle, yet profound, had happened to me that night.

Since that evening in November 1976, the superbrilliant light experience and the quickening phenomena have rarely occurred. But I noticed not long ago the beginning of the original flashing pattern, the same as the one that began in February 1976. Perhaps another cycle has begun.

Before leaving this section on meditation, there is one subject that should be covered — the concept of the "shielding" or protection that is needed when one begins to enter expanded states, either through meditation or through induction by a teacher.

Although the outer rational mind may not accept that there are forms of energy (called astral or elemental entities) capable of doing injury or harm, the actual experience of or encounter with such an energy form usually brings a wild-eyed stampede for information on shielding. As I wrote in the section about Eunice as the teacher, my own outer mind refused to take any part in what I felt was sheer paranoia and fantasy concerning this aspect. Even in my beginning Conference work, I gave only lip service to the concept of shielding. First of all, I really did not believe that it was important, and second, I was working primarily with people who considered such thinking sheer childish superstition. Now, however, having been hit twice by such energy fields, I know better.

In my current Conference work, I ask that people consider the concept of protection and shielding not as an aspect of psychic defense but as an aspect of wisdom. The lesson I use comes from the wonderful example of the butterfly.

I have contemplated this life form for hours on end and have many stories to share about it. I see the life cycle of the butterfly as the quintessence of the Transformational Process. Right here, however, I want to focus on one particular aspect of the caterpillar-butterfly transformation, the phase of the chrysalis.

When the caterpillar is ready to begin the process of transmutation of its physical form, it creates, out of its own physical Beingness, the shield or protection necessary for this process. Some species do not actually weave a cocoon but, instead, in some way harden the outer skin to form the chrysalis. In either case, a defense against the ordinary outside elements is necessary while the critical changes are taking place inside. Open a chrysalis and the process of transformation ceases: the caterpillar during transformation will be destroyed by sunlight alone, an energy that did not faze the caterpillar earlier in its natural skin defense.

The analogy to the human Transformational Process is clear. While the human being is in relatively unawakened and unaware stages of development, while it is in the caterpillar phase, the human consciousness is surrounded by a natural shield of energy. When the time for transformation arrives, however, this natural protection or shielding is disrupted or is simply inadequate. One must begin the process of developing a chrysalis, an energy field that buffers what ordinarily did not need to be buffered before. As will be demonstrated in the chapter on techniques, all energy follows thought. Therefore, all that is necessary to develop a protection or shield is to conceive of an energy surrounding the entire body, and give it the qualities of shielding against any action that may disrupt the Transformational Process. The usual teaching is to surround oneself with white light. Other techniques can be used, but I think this simplest, most familiar approach is often the most effective.

Note that when the process of transformation is complete — after the butterfly is fully developed — the need for the chrysalis ceases. The butterfly emerges, ready to explore a new dimension of Beingness. Similarly, when the Transformational Process is completed in a person, conscious shielding is no longer required.

In conclusion, I must point out that no one can say which of the paths or techniques of meditation is the ''correct'' approach. I definitely do not know. I intuitively feel that every technique can be valuable, but only in relation to the present needs and to the state of development of each individual. One must honor the moment of one's Beingness as it is and deal less with specific details than with the general, constant intention, clearly set, to rise to more inclusive states of action and awareness.

There is an old axiom in medicine: if there are many

treatments for a disease, it is because no one knows much about that disease. I suspect that the same axiom is true for meditation. Whatever method works for you, follow it, and have the courage to say no to a teacher, inner or outer, when it doesn't.

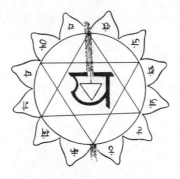

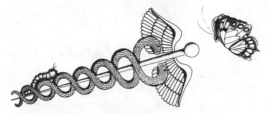

CHAPTER NINE

Departure from Orthodox Medicine, Disease and Death as Transformations, the Transformational Therapist

A problem can never be resolved at the level of the problem, nor a paradox at the level of the paradox. One must rise above the level of the problem or the paradox to find a resolution.

I would like to share with you a set of experiences that, together, formed a pivot in my life. The set contains the final link that allowed my awareness to comprehend a series of dynamics that, in turn, culminated in the sweeping changes in my life in mid-1974.

I have already told you I had known at seventeen that I would not be practicing conventional medicine after the age of thirty-five. The knowledge seemed paradoxical to me. I so thoroughly enjoyed the practice of medicine that I could not imagine any other equally satisfying mode of expressing my Beingness. As it turned out, the event that precipitated the changes did not care about my personal desires or my immediate satisfactions. It was concerned with much deeper commitments.

On January 27, 1974, I turned thirty-five. (If you are interested in astrology, my birthplace was Salt Lake City, Utah,

203

and the hour was 3:00 P.M.) On that day I expected some big, dramatic change; but my morning meditation was nothing special, no beam of golden light split the heavens to illuminate my consciousness, and my birthday celebration — with my twin brother, his wife and my parents, at a Mexican restaurant in Costa Mesa, California — was quiet and undramatic. The only high was induced by a giant margarita.

By the end of the day, however, I had completely rationalized away the intuitive knowledge that I had had for so many years. After all, my life had changed considerably since I had met Eunice and, after her death, the Inner Teacher. I had conceived Command Therapy and was using it in my practice. My exploration of the energy fields of the body was developing rapidly. I was instructing some interested patients and a few physicians in body-energy fields, and in my home each week I met with a group of ten to twelve people to probe more deeply the dream states and the images that can arise in awareness during group meditation. "Perhaps I am already fulfilling the prophesy in some such way that I need not leave orthodox medicine," I thought. The idea eased my mind. I was on my way up in the administrative echelons of the hospital staff. I had had an eighteen-month experience as codirector of medical education on the hospital administrative staff. My working relationships were, in general, excellent. I suspected — and hoped — that I would be able to influence conventional medicine the easy way, from the inside. That evening, in short, I thought that I was going to accomplish my revealed work without having to give anything up. I decided to live in the best of two worlds.

My bliss was the bliss of ignorance. A more fundamental portion of my consciousness had other plans. In this framework I was to learn the consequences of my own immaturity and of my attachment to the ideas I had constructed about my life.

Several months before my thirty-fifth birthday, I had begun to feel a pattern of abdominal pains. They were episodic and, initially, appeared at intervals of about six weeks. The sensation, in the upper abdomen, was a sudden, intense cramping that then radiated to the back; associated with it were nausea, sweating, lightheadedness and weakness. The intensity took only minutes to develop, then remained at the same level for twelve to twenty-four hours. A stoic type, I refused to allow my body to interfere with my commitments, whether to patients or to ideals. Each day of pain, I would finish my professional work, return home, turn the electric blanket to its highest setting and try to sleep. By morning the pain was usually beginning to wane, and after several days I would feel fine, as if the attack had never taken place. I told my wife that I had much greater sympathy for women with menstrual cramping, because my first three attacks were exactly "on schedule." But by February, shortly after my thirty-fifth birthday, the attacks were coming more frequently, about three weeks apart.

Being a diagnostician, I had already surmised that the disease process involved either the pancreas or the small bowel or both. By late March, two months after my thirty-fifth birthday, the attacks were coming every two weeks, and I put myself and my disease into the hands of a specialist in gastrointestinal disorders. After X rays, blood and urine studies and a direct, inside view of my stomach and duodenum by means of fiber optics, he concluded that I was suffering from chronic relapsing pancreatitis. Since all the treatable causes of the disease had been eliminated from our consideration, there was no cure in my case.

From my medical training I knew that the disease is unpredictable. Since it sometimes ends abruptly for an indefinite period of time, each attack can be the last. At the other extreme, each attack can turn it into fulminating pancreatitis, the mortality of which is about 80 percent. In its most common course it leads progressively to pancreatic insufficiency and myriad associated problems.

I tried a deep psychological probe of myself. Why was I manifesting a disease process that could severely restrict my activities or take me out of this plane altogether? The Inner Teacher offered no answer, not even a hint. With each attack, I explored the circumstances that surrounded it, trying to find some pattern; I found none. I examined the stresses in my life, but they were inconsequential in comparison to the disease process and thus not powerful enough to lead to it. I talked to my body, trying to find some symbolic aspect that a malfunctioning pancreas might reflect, but nothing appeared. I simply could not see the dynamics of my problem.

In July 1974 in Los Angeles, I gave my first public lecture. It was for the annual conference of the Center for the Healing Arts, and its title was "Metaphysics, Meditation, and Medicine." In it I shared my experience of dramatic healings in my own work by giving people options to chronic or terminal diseases. By then, five months after my birthday, I was having attacks every three days. I could share my experiences in my patients' cures, but I seemed completely unable to do anything for myself.

The months of July and August kept me very busy. With one or the other of my partners vacationing, my workload was more than doubled. Now my morning meditation was at 4:00 A.M. I arrived at the hospital by 5:30 to begin rounds, and sometimes visited as many as thirty-five hospital patients before 9:30, when I began to see scheduled patients in my office. If there were no emergencies, the workday went on till 10:00 or 11:00 P.M. I loved it.

Then came the thirty minutes that were to alter my entire life.

It was a Saturday morning. I had finished rounds at the hospital and was working on some patients' charts in my office when I felt an incredibly strong urge to enter into meditation. It was so strong that I did not understand what was happening to me. I completed the patients' charts and gave in to the impress. A vortex of energy, of a magnitude I had never before experienced, reverberated through my body and threw my awareness into a superheightened state. Then a loud voice — not that of the Inner Teacher — said, in essence: "Your experience and training as an orthodox physician is completed. It's over. The time has come for you to embark on a rededication of your Beingness to a deeper commitment and action." Automatically my "yes, but" tape came on: "Yes, but can't you see that I am committed to my patients, to my partners, to insurance agents, to the banks, to the IRS, to . . . ?"

The voice didn't care about my many personal concerns and commitments. It next presented to my awareness that I would soon begin a journey into the world, going first to Findhorn and to England, Egypt, India, Nepal near the Tibetan border and perhaps to Japan. This journey was to reawaken old soul memories. They in turn would bring to my awareness knowledge not then available to my outer mind. The voice explained clearly that my vision of being a physician had been distorted by boyhood ideals and by the current concepts of science and medicine, which overemphasized the body and external causes and ignored the journey of the soul. I was to begin the study of alternative healing practices and reach insights Western medicine had not yet dared to dream, insights that would unify exoteric and esoteric traditions and thus form the basis of an integrated approach to the art of healing. The last instruction the voice gave me was simply to detach from everything.

The experience sounds messianic, and it was! In fact, the meditation is as vivid in my mind today as the day it occurred more than four years ago. When one begins to touch upon a collective force greater than one's personal power, the experience is awesome. If the ego or personal level of consciousness claims the more expanded levels as its own, the consequent inflation of ego may be devastating to the self later when the expanded levels are in some way withdrawn or unavailable.

I also realize that the collective areas of awareness influence many different people about the same time. I had a choice of responding to the collective impress or of remaining within the confines of my own personal ego structure. There are many other people whose study of alternative healing practices will lead to insights Western medicine has not yet seen. They, too, will have an opportunity to integrate exoteric and esoteric traditions. Like seeds scattered upon the earth, some will come to fruition and many will not. In my case, the choice was and still is whether to participate in a more universal pattern of life or to remain within personal systems of thought and action. Fortunately, my ego structure is able to allow expanded impresses to function through me without confusing the collective and the individual selves.

I knew that the voice had spoken deep truths. I saw the reawakened vision. Everything I had established materially — financial security, possessions, professional reputation, social status, even friends and family — was to be left behind. For exactly what, I did not know, but I did know, by the time the meditation was over, that I felt a connection to the deepest level of my Beingness. I was entrusting the course of my life to a Higher Orchestrator. By the end of those thirty minutes, I had surrendered.

On coming out of that meditation, I dictated my resignation from my partnership and letters requesting leaves of absence from the hospital staff and my academic teaching positions, called a realtor to put the house up for sale and asked a friend to sell the cars. Wendey was traveling at the time. When I finally reached her, she was excited by my meditation experience but was not entirely convinced that I would really carry out such a vast change in my life.

In six weeks everything was gone — practice, teaching positions, home, cars and most of the furnishings and clothes. Before the meditation I had never heard of Findhorn, but I soon learned that it was a spiritual community in northern Scotland. If the vortex that swept over me was like the tornado that carried Dorothy and Toto to the Land of Oz, my Yellow Brick Road began at Findhorn.

(If you cannot accept the idea of the voice because you do not understand it, I fully sympathize with you. You will find it even more difficult to believe that the voice spoke to me of Findhorn, of which I had never heard. I do not understand the voice, either, and I cannot explain — in any brief, easily comprehensible terms, in terminology accessible to the rational outer mind — how the voice could talk about things I had never heard of. But I accept both the voice and what the voice said. And, of course, I have a further advantage: I *know* it happened.)

In the six weeks before leaving for Europe, I lived in two simultaneous feeling states, pain and exhilaration. My pain was associated with detaching myself from loved ones, patients, a home that inspired me every time I returned to it, a stimulating lifestyle and the security that surrounded it all. On the other side, the exhilaration of leaping into the unknown was intoxicating. My future no longer offered a single set of possibilities, as predictable as the social, cultural and material artifacts from which they stemmed. My life was now filled with a great number of sets of possibilities, infinitely varied. I felt a new sense of vitality rising from the roots of my being. The wellspring that nourished my awareness was the knowing — the absolute *knowing* — that the course of the action I was following was true to my soul. The jump off the cliff into what appeared to be oblivion simply didn't matter.

I barely remember the six to eight weeks before I arrived in Scotland. My outer mind was dazzled. It was not until the second day there, while I was walking along the North Sea coast, that I suddenly woke up to reality.

I had not had a single attack of abdominal pain since the morning of the meditation.

"Of course."

No other words were possible, because the insight was clear: the intensity of energy that reverberated through my body during the transformational meditation healed the chronic relapsing pancreatitis totally, completely and instantaneously. My disease had been the signal of a major force within me that was demanding change. There had been a choice to follow either my outer mind or my soul. I had chosen my soul's path, and my soul was free to flow.

Until the time of the great meditation, my outer mind had completely rationalized its position on conventional medicine — in fact, on everything about my life. But the deeper pattern and path had been there all the time. I just hadn't wanted to look at them. And my refusal to look at them had been part of the "cause" of the disease.

I had already learned much in my work with cancer patients. If a disease is on a terminating or downhill course, a Transformational Process is manifesting. The obvious transformation toward which that person is heading is physical death, but there may also be a transformation on this side, in the living. If that transformation is chosen and if it is to be effective, the change in the patient's attitudes and life patterning must be as complete as would transpire through death. Halfway means won't do it; there is no room for compromise. Sweeping changes are required, and each individual knows what those changes must be. Marshaling the courage and clarity to make the necessary changes is the real challenge.

The vaster area of our Beingness does not know what death or disease is. Not that this vaster area is simply ignorant. Quite the contrary. It is the outer, fragmented aspects of our Beingness that are ignorant; they do not realize the consequences of focusing our awareness on conditioned ideas about life and values. When change is called for—often by a disease process or some other serious disruption in one's life—we have a choice; we can take the direct action that will harmonize our Beingness, or we can block ourselves from that direct action and let our outer minds pretend that we don't understand. Our disease or our psychological knot is doing for us what we couldn't or wouldn't do directly and with awareness. When our outer mind cannot or will not manifest the essence of our desire, the unconscious mechanism does it for us. Without our understanding it or willing it, the unconscious mechanism finds a pathway out of the mode from which the psyche desires release. The path it finds may not be to the liking of the outer mind, such as death to the cancer or pancreatitis patient; but it is nevertheless, like death, an effective way out. If the action of the mind obstructs the soul from fulfilling its fundamental life commitments, then mental diseases, emotional disorders and diseases of the body ensue. On the other hand, transformation brings about resolution. One way or the other, through cure or through death, it resolves the symptoms and the disease.

This personal Transformational Process is the foundation of all my work, both with individual clients and with Conference participants. The principles involved in the unblocking of the soul's flow can be applied universally. In this widespread sense they are the basis of a psycho-physical-spiritual therapeutic interaction called Transformational Psychology. The word *psychology*, literally interpreted, *is* the study of the soul, even though current usage restricts it almost entirely to the outer mind. Transformational Psychology is nothing less than the study of the transformation of the soul — the freeing of the soul into natural expression. Its fundamental focus in the treatment of the human being is the mind that has somehow walked into a closet, closed the door, turned out the light and instantly forgotten all these events.

Most conventional therapeutic approaches to the mind now recognize the mind-body relationship, but hardly any of them accept experientially the body-mind-soul integrity. A mind cut off from the very source of its essence, the soul, is like a body cut off from its brain. In coma, or when portions of the brain are destroyed through anoxia, trauma or destructive disease processes, the body still functions to a very limited degree and can be viable for long periods of time; but it is never anywhere near to complete functioning. In a similar way, the mind cut off from the soul is viable and can function in very limited degrees. Clearly, the soul that animates the mind is analogous to the mind that animates the body. When all three are in conjunction, the Transformational Process of the human being is greatly accelerated.

From the metaphysical perspective, a person's body is essentially "perfect" for that individual in any particular lifetime. There may be certain "built-in" restrictions that act to limit a particular person's physical or mental actions, but, no matter how the outer mind conceives of them, these restrictions are always for the betterment of the individual. Once the individual accepts the limitation — and turns to the development of other resources — the limitation has served its purpose and is no longer necessary in this or later lifetimes. The individual is enriched through the limitation. In any individual the soul is always the most advanced aspect, at a developmental stage far, far beyond the awareness of the outer mind or the body.

It is the outer mind, with its memories, that causes the

difficulties. The outer awareness often ignores the covenant with the body. It goes off in its constructs of reality and treats the body as no more than an object. But the mind's constructs are developed by way of highly filtered perceptions, and it is the mind, not the body, that blocks spiritual awareness. The body and the spirit need no education. It is the outer mind, in relationship to the soul, that is undergoing the training and the experiences in this dimension. The mind, which ought to be the liaison between the physical and the spiritual, is the only aspect of the human being that has to be integrated. Of the three, the mind is the only portion that can be confused!

There are no such things as spiritual confusions or body confusions — only mind confusions. Once the mind capitulates to the higher essence, psychological diseases (confusion) and most diseases caused by the mind's interaction with the body simply disappear.

The soul is an individuation out of spirit. The mind, as we unconventionally conceive it here, is essentially a byproduct, an observer — that is, until it tries to usurp the place of the soul and the body, and then it creates pandemonium. From the spiritual perspective, the mind must be continually reminded that the body is an energy configuration of the soul-spirit interaction — with the mind as a witness. Mind in the usual sense of the word does not create the body, though it would often like to think that it does, nor does the mind create the soul, as it very often thinks it does. The mind is not and cannot be dominant in the mind-body-soul triad. It is the mind's attempts to be dominant that cause most of our problems in this plane.

Transformational Psychology is a tool to integrate the three parts of the triad. Recognizing that the patient's mind, with its memory bank of experiences both in this lifetime and in many prior lifetimes, is what makes all the mistakes, Transformational Psychology places direct responsibility for physical and psychological disease directly upon the patient, specifically upon the patient's mind. The true reality of the soul-and-body relationship, from which the mind is only a byproduct, is literally mind-boggling: it is simply incomprehensible and intolerable to the intellect. Until the mind can accept this status and reposition itself to become the soul's witness on the physical plane, pain and suffering remain. Once the mind accepts that the soul's consciousness and awareness transcend the consciousness and awareness of the mind itself, there is freedom. One no longer needs to remain within the confines of the outer mind.

Transformational Psychology recognizes three stages in any Transformational Process. First is the awakening to the realization that most of the experiences of life perceived as external to oneself are actually projections of the self onto reality. The second stage emphasizes the "owning" of these projections—pulling them back into the individual's mind and integrating them with the concept of self. This stage is the critical one. In it one must learn that the dynamics of any problem are clearly under one's own power and control and therefore changeable or, in a term of Transformational Psychology, transmutable. This second stage is completed when what is really "out there" can be perceived without distortion. In the final Transformational Process, one knows that there is no separation between what is experienced as external and what is experienced as internal; they are the same thing. There is no external or internal reality to distinguish.

The Tibetan Buddhist approach to the resolution of problems delineates three pathways. The highest and most difficult is to transmute the problem—that is, to generate an intensity of energy from a higher, more expanded awareness and to use this energy to force a change in the configuration of the problem's less expanded, less intense energy and thus to free the energy that configurates the problem. Transmutation implies a change of the form or nature (of anything) into another form or nature. In this plane, all energy flows from more energetic sources to less energetic manifestations, never in the opposite direction. Therefore, higher aspects of consciousness always transmute lower aspects of consciousness.

The second Tibetan Buddhist pathway is to ennoble the problem, to treat it as a necessary and important steppingstone of experience in one's unfolding. In the West, this process is called rationalization, and it has a negative connotation rather than the positive insight that it has from the Buddhist viewpoint.

The third Tibetan Buddhist pathway is to go directly into the problem and allow it to manifest completely. There is but one injunction: one must make a portion of one's awareness into a witness that observes the problem. In this way, understanding may come. This last method is considered to be the path of subtle wisdom, and for many people it is a more appropriate pathway than that of direct transmutation. In practice, most of us use various combinations of the three pathways in dealing with our personal problems.

Vitvan, a Western mystic, taught that there were two ways of dealing with problems. One was to transmute the problem, and the second was to wear it out! Sometimes it seems that most of us are stuck with the latter method.

Transformational Psychology does not try to make any individual "normal." Instead, its approach is based on the realization that in this lifetime each individual is working out certain aspects of development on a far vaster scale than that of most psychotherapeutic modalities. For example, one individual may be developing deeper resources in the mental area, with less emphasis on the sexual and the emotional areas, while another individual may be working on the development of emotional expression and not the mental or sexual. I consider it absurd to believe that every soul is to be "integrated" into a "normal," "healthy" pattern. No two human beings are working on exactly the same developments at the same time. Until the therapist's consciousness can embrace the continuity of Life—can accept that the soul of the individual is in a developmental process requiring many dimensions of experience — most psychotherapeutic work, misunderstanding the life process, becomes an awkward coercion toward uninspired uniformity — or, even worse, toward a self-centered commonality.

Why must we continually learn about our immortality through the process called death? When are we going to awaken into our immortality while living? When are we going to give up the concept of the "innocent victim"? When will we realize that disease is simply doing for us what we ourselves refuse to do? Why must we generate the energy of crisis to approach the spiritual? Transformational Psychology shifts the perspective of the outer mind toward these questions.

I wish to state honestly that the development of Transformational Psychology as a therapeutic approach is only in its beginning stages. It is not a polished product, nor is it by any means complete. The premises, though not experimentally proved, are experientially sound. Finally, there are, at most, ten or twelve people who are practicing this or a similar form of therapy.

The Transformational therapist, already in the process of working through the filters of his or her own mind, is at a stage of not only clearly seeing the outer mind of the client, but also entering telepathically into a rapport with the client's soul and thus gaining insight into the particular dynamics that that soul is expressing. Thus, the Transformational therapist is in contact with the flow not only of his or her own soul, but of the patient's soul as well. This particular development of the therapist comes through the meditative process, through working with a teacher or through both.

The Transformational therapist has developed the ability to heighten his or her own consciousness at will. The heart-chakra center, and usually the throat center, the forehead center and the crown center are functioning in a more refined state than in ordinary states of awareness. Again, this control over the chakras of the therapist is achieved through a meditative process, with the help of the heightening influence of the teacher.

The Transformational therapist realizes that the client is a mirror to the therapist's own consciousness and that the therapist is a mirror for the client as well. The therapist tries not to forget that the dynamics the client is working through have equivalent counterparts in his or her own consciousness. The therapist, working with the client's dynamics, is working with the identical dynamics in himself or herself at the same time.

As is implicit from our earlier discussion of the hologram,

the Transformational therapist is capable of a state of consciousness in which he or she knows that the totality of his or her own Beingness contains the Beingness of the client. Without the client's having to express it in any way—physically, emotionally or verbally—the therapist's consciousness contains everything there is to know about the client. The therapist is aware, too, that in the same way the client has the potential of knowing all that the therapist represents and senses.

Initially, the Transformational therapist may use such clues as voice vibration, body language and the emotional responses of the client to help guide his or her personal consciousness to the area that reflects the client. At a later stage of the therapist's development these clues are no longer necessary. The therapist experiences the client directly.

Realizing that the specific problem of the client is only the shadow of a much deeper pattern dynamic, the Transformational therapist does not start at the problem level, the level at which the client perceives the difficulty. Instead, the Transformational therapist tries to comprehend the pattern level of consciousness, which is manifesting the "problem," and to focus the transmutational energy there. Nothing of much value—perhaps nothing of *any* value—will happen if the client's awareness is allowed to remain in the perspective of the problem. Clients are so conditioned to play their tragedy records, repeating their problems over and over again not only to therapists, but to almost anybody who will listen, that if they stay on the problem level they are almost certain to continue to play the same song over and over forever in an endless groove.

The first task of the Transformational therapist, then, is to heighten the client's awareness into a state of clarity. This opening process can be accomplished by several techniques. One way is simply to ignore the problem. The more the client attempts to amplify it, the more the therapist is to ignore the amplification and to avoid interaction with it. The client may rant and cry, scream and act out, and all of it is to be ignored. If a quiet meditation with the client doesn't work, the therapist may resort to getting the client to dance, to going swimming with the client, to telling an outrageous joke inducing laughter, to taking a walk with the client, to doing T'ai Chi, to singing or to chanting with the client—anything to shift the perspective of the client away from the problem level in the outer mind. The actual heightening of the client's awareness comes about through an induction process. The therapist's level of consciousness, as reflected through his or her body fields, induces a similar level of consciousness in the client's energy field, and the client's consciousness shifts concomitantly to form an appropriate fit to the new energy field. Induction is the process by which a body having electric or magnetic properties produces magnetism, an electric charge or an electromotive force in a neighboring body, without contact. Until the client releases the perspective from the problem level, therapeutic interaction is not possible. Energy-field induction through the heart chakra, manifesting a state of Unconditional Love, lifts the client up, out of the level the outer mind is configurating as the problem, into a state of clarity. If the Transformational therapist is in a state of Unconditional Love, and if induction occurs, the client *cannot* stay at the problem level.

The Transformational therapist may have to work directly with the client's chakras. In this technique, energy is transferred through the therapist's hands to induce the shift in the client's awareness. (This part of the work will be discussed in the chapter on techniques.)

Once the client is in a heightened state of consciousness, the Transformational therapist induces the witness state. In it, the client can see the problem level without reacting to it either mentally or emotionally. When all the options are seen simultaneously, the client's evaluation will shift automatically to the pattern level. Since the options seen in the heightened state of consciousness may be overwhelming when the client's emotional and mental levels are reintegrated later, the therapist must carefully prepare the client for this possibility.

If the client accepts the options and the new value system envisioned in the heightened state of awareness, the problem or disease configuration will alter in direct relationship to the client's commitment to a new course of action and to his or her ability to sustain that action. The therapist can assume no responsibility for it. The commitment and the sustaining of that commitment are entirely the responsibility of the client.

While the therapist and the client are together in the heightened state of awareness, the therapist brings out as much of the totality of the client's Beingness as the client is capable of experiencing. Instead of continuing on with what he or she thinks is his or her purpose and intention in this lifetime, the client must learn to perceive the intention of his or her soul. This area is where Transformational Psychology becomes an art, and where the therapist must be not a scientist or metaphysician, not an advisor or counselor, but an artist.

When it is necessary, the Transformational therapist is able to help a dying client through physical death. The choice is always the client's. Transformation on through death is one and the same thing as the Transformational Process in life. As you may realize, it is only the prejudiced, conditioned outer mind that sees the one transformation as different from the other.

The Transformational therapist teaches the client to be able to induce the heightened state of awareness for himself or herself. The techniques include the use of a piece of music that is conditioned to the therapeutic interaction (this method will be discussed in depth in the next chapter); practice of the spiral-meditation technique; and the playing of a tape recording of the therapeutic session. These techniques, whether in combination or alone, tend to place the client's consciousness in a level similar to that of the session.

It is impossible to overemphasize the value of tape recordings of therapeutic sessions. Because of the phenomenon of state-bound consciousness, the client cannot remember, even for a few hours, what the critical areas of resolution were. This forgetting does not occur only in Transformational experiences, but is, in general, common in any kind of psychotherapeutic exchange. Though one rarely hears of people recording their sessions with their analysts, I feel strongly that they should insist on doing so. I am sure that many problems would be resolved much more quickly.

During the course of the interaction, the Transformational therapist can work with any significant dream material that the client may offer. The purpose is not to interpret the dream but to teach the client the relationship of the inner dream to the outer reality, because this relationship always reveals the pattern level of consciousness.

Toward the close of the initial therapeutic interaction, the therapist reminds the client that the client's awareness may be repolarized back into the problem perspective. The experienced Transformational therapist may even choose to demonstrate this possibility by deliberately inducing the problem level and then inducing the resolution level, so that the client can experience the dramatic shift in awareness and feeling states that the repolarization process engenders.

At the close of the session, the Transformational therapist impresses on the client the beauty and magnificence of the Life process and the opening up of opportunities for personal development presented by the "problem." The client, inspired and uplifted, senses that he or she is beginning to manifest the highest potential available.

I oppose the usual, habitual practices of an hour's interaction and of daily or weekly meetings. A minimum of three hours or even an entire day may be necessary to work fully into and out of a Transformational experience. The therapist also discourages the dependence of the client by seeing the client infrequently, perhaps at six-week intervals, or monthly at the most.

Last, the Transformational therapist knows when to do absolutely nothing for a client—probably the most difficult aspect to master in a "do-something-do-anything" society.

What is most to be deplored is any technique or any medication that allows the patient simply to *cope* with life. Nobody wants just to cope, everyone wants more. When the client is precipitated into heightened states of resolution, the symptoms of anxiety, depression and fear dissolve. While tranquilizers and other "therapeutic" drugs only mask the symptoms that have been functioning as signals to tell the outer mind that change is necessary, the transformation of the client's value systems is real therapy. It *is* change.

The frequent or habitual use of mind-expanding drugs by either the therapist or the client also works against the psychotherapeutic interaction. Although the drug experience can be a breakthrough for an individual, continued use of psychedelics, hallucinogens or other drugs eventually blocks the ability, in either the therapist or the client, to achieve natural expanded states of awareness. From personal exploration with hallucinogens, I know that the drug experience is less satisfactory and less productive than naturally induced higher states of awareness.

In exploring Transformational Psychology in Conferences at Sky Hi Ranch, I have found that the heightening process and the development of overview are accelerated by the group experience. The energy field of a group is far more intense than that of a Transformational therapist alone. Control of the group field is vital to success, however, because if the group is precipitated into negative or contracted states, the therapist must use every resource of his or her Beingness to recenter the group.

The most crucial factor in the use of Transformational Psychology is the level of development of the therapist. No matter how thoroughly trained his or her outer mind may be, it must never direct the psychotherapeutic interaction. However highly developed, it is still the outer mind, too limited to be allowed control. It is not to be the dominant orchestrator but, at best, a useful and important tool.

Not all clients are able to allow the induction into higher states of awareness. We must keep in mind that, while the outer mind is not the source of the problem, it invariably compounds the problem. Since the problem level always serves clients in secondary ways, they may be unwilling or unable to relinquish their attachment to it. As a rule I find that if a client, after the therapeutic session, repolarizes the problem quickly, he or she is hanging on to the problem with great intensity; if the problem is repolarized slowly, the client is on the way to being able to let the problem level go.

In the psychotherapeutic interaction it is usually desirable that the client be sufficiently intelligent to comprehend what is happening during the session, but intelligence is certainly not essential. When the mind is incapable of understanding the process, the induction from the therapist's energy fields to the client's fields often brings comprehension by itself. The client may not know *what* has happened, but he or she will certainly be aware that *something* has happened.

Psychoses are not beyond the reach of Transformational Psychology, but their treatment requires a very high development on the part of the therapist. The therapist must not only transmute his or her own fear of psychosis, but must also understand the psychotic process, because psychosis is not necessarily an abnormal state. Violent clients can be treated, but only by a therapist whose energy fields are intense. Obviously, extreme cases require incarceration, hospitalization or both until the crisis subsides. During the crisis, however, the Transformational therapist can still continue with induction work, sometimes with dramatic effect.

The therapist must realize that when a client is on a self-destructive course, the therapeutic approach may be *not* to interfere with it. Always, what determines the proper therapeutic procedure is not the desires of society or of an individual therapist's outer conditioned mind or of the expecting part of the client's mind. The key is the flow of the soul. The therapist's task is to determine where the soul is going and then to help clear away the blocks to its getting there.

In our age of transition, we shall witness the blending of the medical, the scientific and the psychospiritual approaches in the healing spectrum available to all human beings.

We are already on the way.

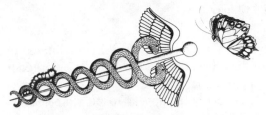

CHAPTER TEN

Exercises and Techniques

*All energy flowing in and
around the body can be directed by thought.*

The two fundamental skills in Transformational Therapy are the
ability to feel body-energy fields and the ability to transfer
heart-chakra energy. To develop these skills, I teach seven
different categories of exercises:

1. The Resonation Circle
2. The exploration of greatly amplified musical sounds
3. The modified spiral meditation
4. Dyadic exercises
5. Triadic exercises
6. Hand scanning
7. Energy transfer

Except for two of the dyadic exercises—the basic eye
exercise (Trespasso technique), from a John Lilly workshop,
and the shield-penetration exercise Eileen Pittler (Weiner)

shared in a workshop she and I cofacilitated in March 1976—
all of these exercises and techniques emerged from the intuitive
area of my consciousness.

The exercises appear to be simple, but each should be
mastered before the student moves on to the next. Not one of the
techniques is unimportant in developing the body-energy control necessary to the conscious sharing of one's energies with
another. They should not be performed immediately after a
meal; they are best performed several hours after a meal.

Most people can learn to do a hand scan in five minutes.
Many can learn to focus energy through the hands in five
minutes. But without much more background, the quality and
the control of that energy is lacking. When it is focused, the
energy with which people work can be as destructive to the body
as it can be healing and harmonizing. When you are working
with a partner or in a triangle, it is your responsibility to deliver
as highly refined an energy as possible. Ignorance is no excuse.
It is your responsibility to know—or, if you do not know, to
learn—before you practice.

When teaching body-energy techniques to participants in
Conferences, I clearly point out in my initial remarks that the
constant focus of attention on the heart-chakra level produces a
temporary distortion of the body-energy fields. The heart-
chakra energy field, accentuated, temporarily becomes the predominant energy radiation from the body.

The body area corresponding to each chakra reflects a
specific level of awareness and has associated with it localized
bodily sensations. Clairvoyants and persons trained to detect
body-energy fields through their hands can easily determine
the predominant state of consciousness of any individual by
determining which energy field is most active at a given moment. For example, intellectual activity stimulates primarily the
forehead-chakra field, emotional states are reflected primarily
in an increase in the radiation of the solar-plexus and splenic
chakras and sexual responses are first seen in the lower-
abdominal chakra.

These radiations have counterparts in the feelings experienced by the subject. Whether a thought activates a certain chakra, or whether stimulation of a certain chakra initiates particular thoughts in that level of awareness, there is always a linking between the individual's awareness and the radiations from his or her corresponding chakra. If a person is radiating primarily from the emotional chakra, his or her perception of all external events will be distorted toward the emotional. An individual primarily in a sexual state of arousal will tend to perceive external stimuli as sexual.

This tendency of consciousness to be interlinked with a specific chakra, to match its perspective, led to the device of having students deliberately focus attention on the heart chakra in order to stimulate this center and thus begin to experience reality from this perspective. The Transformational Process is intimately connected with the heart-chakra level of awareness.

Before proceeding any further, it is necessary to clarify the matter of the quality of the energy fields radiating from the chakras.

All chakras function actively in all individuals, alive or dead, as long as the body is configurated in human form. I must emphasize, most strongly, that an active chakra is not necessarily an *awakened* or *developed* chakra. The intensity of a chakra field does not indicate that it is developed but only that it is functioning. The level of functioning of a specific chakra is determined by the *quality* of the energy emerging from the chakra. This quality is reflected in the color seen clairvoyantly or in the frequency felt by hand scanning and, in addition, in the configuration of the emitted field. An unawakened crown chakra, for example, may be intense but undeveloped, its field shaped more like a cylinder than like the plume or cone that is detected in individuals with awakened crown energies. The same holds true for all major chakras of the body. I can say it briefly now, but it took me three years to understand this simple differentiation.

Sexual energy can be transmuted into emotional energy, mental energy or physical energy. The same is true of all so-called primary responses of the human being. The human being has options available to no other life form on this planet except, perhaps, the dolphin. Yet, because of the relatively undeveloped awareness of human beings (even the most highly developed intellect is only a fragment of the individual's total awareness), hardly anyone realizes that these options exist, and experiential awareness of them is even rarer.

The transmutational process operates subconsciously in most people today. It is this subconscious operation and its conflict with the underdeveloped state of the outer awareness that create the knots in the human psyche and result in physical, emotional and mental aberrations. If people understood the basic mechanisms of awareness, there would be no such thing as repressed anger, sexuality, hostility and so on.

The present state of consciousness of the human being is intolerable. If no higher aspect were available, humanity would be better off returning to the natural simplicity of animal consciousness. In my optimism, however, I sense that the current unacceptable state of human awareness is, though it has been this way for at least fifteen or twenty thousand years, only transitional. Today we are on the brink of a new era, there is a choice, and the choice is ours. We cannot know whether our conditioned awareness has been developed because of or in spite of intelligence, but we can and must choose either to continue to manifest that awareness, the transitional primate awareness, or to claim aspects of our Divinity.

The magnificence of the heart perspective of awareness is the direct connection to the Divine aspects. There is only one other direct connection with the Divine, that through the crown chakra, a later natural development, available usually only after the heart chakra develops or unfolds.

To help bring about the connection to the Divine, the Conference participant is asked to hold sexual, emotional, mental and physical chakras in check and express his or her energies only through the heart chakra until he or she experiences the options available through the perspective of the heart chakra.

An angry person, for example, discovers that chronic anger is energy distorted into a destructive way of expression. That person learns that the energy of this destructive distortion can be transmuted if it is expressed through the heart chakra. With this understanding of the transmutation, one can begin to see that the anger has, really, little to do with the event that "precipitated" it but is inextricably connected with one's own distorted and overly sensitive emotional chakra, with its predisposition to react to certain experiences with anger. When an angry person comes to see that there is an alternative to reacting toward certain stimuli with anger—whether or not he or she ever actually uses that alternative—that person is waking up.

When an individual dominated by sexual energy discovers that this secondary energy need not be released in this habitual way, that there are options in the transmutation of sexual energy by way of alternative chakras, that human being is awakening.

The key is not blocking experiences—not necessarily stopping the anger or the sexuality in our examples—but having options in any experience. The Divine aspect of humanity is the ability to choose without distortion. One effect of the full awakening of an individual's awareness is the mastery of the choice of expression and experience. With this mastery, distortions of the sexual, the emotional, the physical and the mental areas of awareness are dissipated, and at last it is possible to experience—singly or in combination, as in a Bach fugue—the purely physical, the purely sexual, the purely emotional, and the purely mental. The Divine human emerges.

THE RESONATION CIRCLE

Energy work during a Conference begins at the first meal. The participants are asked to join hands before they begin to eat. At this point they are asked only to let go of mental and emotional concerns, to focus their attention on their lower chest, to bring in feelings of inspiration and harmony and to share these feelings with everyone at the table. The dining area is so arranged that all the participants and I sit at two or three large tables connected together. Our circle of hands, called "the resonation," becomes an essential exercise and the one most often repeated during the Conference. Before each meal, and at the beginning and end of each session held in the seminar room, a resonation is performed so that it is experienced at least seven times a day. By the fourth day of a Conference, the energy of the group usually reaches such intensity that few are unaware of the power of this interaction.

During the first session of the Conference, I discuss the importance of the resonation exercise. In the Conference room the participants sit in a circle on large pillows on the floor. Most sit cross-legged, but any position that allows them to hold hands comfortably is adequate. I introduce into the circle a simple biofeedback device that sends an imperceptible charge of electricity through the entire group when they are holding hands. It makes a sound as long as the contact remains unbroken, and the pitch of the sound varies with the electrical resistance in the circuit. It demonstrates quickly and easily, first, that the group is acting as a conduit of energy flow, and, second, that individual members of the group can modify the flow of the current and thus alter the pitch of the sound coming from the instrument. By analogy, we infer that as the participants begin to develop individual "charges" of energy coming from their heart-chakra areas, the "charge" passing through the group as they hold hands is intensified. There is more to the analogy, but what is important is the experience of the resonation circle, not the theory behind it.

In the resonation, the task is always the same: one must center one's awareness on one's heart chakra. I emphasize that just thinking about doing it will begin to make it happen. Begin to direct the energies of the body to the heart area. Once the idea initiates the energy flow, the focus of awareness must be entirely on the heart chakra. *One cannot think about what it would be like to be totally focused in the heart-chakra area*; one must *feel* and *be* the heart chakra. (The first sequence of words in italics are, individually as well as together, totally wrong; the second two words are totally right.)

As the exercise continues, one may feel some sensations in the chest area. There may be a warmth, a thumping (because the heart muscle itself is being stimulated), a tingling, sometimes a vibratory sensation and, infrequently, pain. Pain in the area of a chakra invariably occurs when there is a great concentration of energy without any way to release that energy. I have had men and women in their twenties swear they were having heart attacks. These individual's bodies were simply not accustomed to focusing energy in this area. When they are told to discharge the energy buildup by imaging it flowing out of the heart chakra, perpendicular to the surface of the skin over the heart-chakra area, the pain symptoms subside. Always allow an exit for an energy buildup in any chakra. Simply conceive or im-agine the energy projecting from the body in the area of buildup. The discomfort quickly subsides.

This exercise is basic — to center one's awareness and energy in the heart chakra and image the release of the built-up energy through the chakra, like a beam, sending it straight out from the chest. After a few days, all participants can not only center at the level of the heart chakra, but also bring energy from anywhere in the body to the heart level and express that energy through the heart chakra.

At first the sensation of energy flow is vague. As the exercise is repeated, it becomes a specific sensation. At some point, the awareness of Unconditional Love appears, associated with a wonderful sense of well-beingness. The natural impulse then is to share this sensation and state of consciousness by projecting the energy from the heart chakra to another indi-vidual, to the group as a whole or to family and friends at a distance.

At the beginning, the group energy field is what I call incoherent. The different members' energy fields are at differ-ent intensities and levels of focus. Most predominant are the forehead energies, the solar-plexus energies, and, occasionally, the sexual and the throat energies. Rarely does an individual initially center the body energies at the heart level. The task for all participants is to become primarily centered in the heart chakra and to stay there during the entire conference. Success at this task has consequences, as I will share.

To bring a group into a single frequency—as happens in the resonation exercise when individuals' energies become centered at the heart-chakra level—has some interesting parallels in physics.

Incoherent light—such as light from an incandescent light bulb—is composed of many frequencies of light energy. It is effective, but not nearly as powerful as a single frequency of light emanating from a light source. Light of a single frequency is called coherent light—or the laser beam. Most people are aware of the power of laser light as compared to ordinary light from a light bulb. The situation in group work is analogous. When the energy field of the group becomes coherent—the field at one level only—it becomes intensified, just as laser light does. As William Tiller of Stanford University suggests on the basis of his research work, the intensity of the coherent group-energy field is not the sum of the number of group members but is, instead, the square of the number of people in the group. Thus, the power of a group of 200 people whose energies were coherent would not have the numerical value of 200 but of 40,000! The induction potential of a group field can be very powerful. Furthermore, one or two individuals with strong energy fields centered at the heart level are capable of igniting the rest of the group into that same level of consciousness. Other individuals who aren't quite centered at the heart level are inducted into the coherent frequency of the heart level. One always has the option of breaking or blocking such an action, but I don't know of anybody who would want to.

A word of caution is also in order here. Mass hysteria is engendered by the exact same principles. Anybody who has ever been swept up into one of these experiences knows the overwhelming power of a group of human beings out of control. The same phenomenon occurs to an audience listening to an inspired speaker or to a particularly excellent actor or actress who is able to manipulate the entire audience through this principle. One feels even greater pathos or greater humor because of the group field than one would if there were just oneself and the speaker!

In talking about induction, I am always quickened by a true story, written by Lyall Watson in his introduction to Lawrence Blair's book *Rhythms of Vision*.

A species of monkeys that lived off the coast of Japan, on widely separated islands with no contact among the groups, had been studied by researchers for more than twenty years. After that length of time, there was little that was not known about them.

In addition to food brought to the islands by the observers, the monkeys ate sweet potatoes that grew wild there. For as long as they had been observed, they had been digging them up and eating them, dirt and all.

But one day on one island, an observer saw one monkey dig up a potato. Instead of eating it dirt and all, the monkey took it down to the seashore and washed off the dirt before he ate it. Shortly, he taught his mother to do the same thing. The mother, in turn, taught her mate, and soon most of the monkeys on that island were taking their potatoes down to the water and washing them before they ate them.

So far, the story sounds like something out of an elementary-psychology course, but Watson has more to tell. (Because the exact number is not known, he uses the number 100 symbolically.)

Eventually the hundredth monkey digs up a potato and takes it down to the shore to wash it. Then, most curiously, within an hour after the hundredth monkey washes its potato, monkeys on two other widely separated islands begin to take their potatoes down to the seashore to wash them before they eat them.

The significance of the story excites me. The suggestion that spatial barriers are transcended when cohesive group action reaches a critical level should ignite anyone who participates in prayer circles, healing circles, communes, church groups, meditation groups, in fact, any gathering of people whose main thrust is service to humanity and whose emphasis is on harmony.

Is it possible that the similarity of geographically widely separate forms of architecture—such as the pyramids in Egypt and those of the Americas and Asia—was based on the same phenomenon? Is this kind of energy interaction involved in the nearly simultaneous creative insights that inventors and writers experience? Could small but powerful groups of individuals telepathically influence the general field of human thought? Does the holographic analogy apply to human consciousness? My mind reels—filled with questions and possibilities that support the concept that we are all somehow interconnected.

THE EXPLORATION OF GREATLY AMPLIFED SOUND

A major experience and exercise that can heighten the consciousness of both the individual and the group is the exploration of greatly amplified music. At the beginning of each group session, the participants in a Conference lie on their backs with the palms of their hands touching the floor. They are warned that the music is going to be at an intensity well above the usual listening range. If the sound is too loud, earplugs are available.

The participants center at the heart level and witness what happens to their bodies, especially to the hands and lower chest area during the experience. One side of a carefully chosen record is played. In case there may be adverse reactions, I do not join the group but observe it.

The seminar room has a double-padded carpet, a powerful quadraphonic sound system, a wood planked floor and, under it, a huge basement. The effect is like lying on top of a very large, very loud drum.

The music is selected for its ability to stimulate various areas of the body that, in turn, organize and entrain the energy fields. Selections are chosen primarily from the classics, because I have discovered that most classical composers are masters in the organization of energy, the energy of sound. The effect is that each person's energy field is doing exactly what every other person's energy field is doing at exactly the same time. At an unconscious level, the group is being trained to harmonize energy fields. The process is entirely beyond conscious understanding; it is experienced both physically and psychologically.

The experience of intense musical sound can precipitate confusion, disorientation and pain in the body, regardless of the selection of music; but some selections are far more capable of generating adverse reactions than others. To minimize these reactions, I carefully screen all the music. I am not particularly interested in whether the music is "great" in the aesthetic sense; I am more interested in the effects on the body-energy fields and the stimulation of the image-making areas of the brain associated with unusual states of awareness.

There are a number of physical, emotional and mental reactions that may occur with the music:

1. There may be a sensation of high frequencies centered in and about the head and neck, medium ranges concentrated in the midportion of the body (the chest and upper abdomen) and low frequencies centered in the abdomen and legs. Certain low frequencies may also cause the chest to vibrate.

2. There may be a sensation of harmonizing or integrating various areas of the body, especially with the music of Bach, Beethoven and Mozart.

3. Involuntary movements of the hands, arms and legs may occur. They may be rhythmic or may be intermittent and irregular.

4. At first, the fingers and palms of the hands may be able to sense only certain frequencies. Sometimes there is a marked difference between the sensations in the right hand and those in the left.

5. With the stimulation of the music, body areas that are ordinarily not sensed may emerge into the awareness and create new three-dimensional images of the body.

6. Pains or aches may develop anywhere in the body. They point out areas that are blocked to the energy flow produced by intense musical sound. This reaction helps draw attention to particular areas that need special attention during those meditative exercises that concentrate on energy flow in the body. It is often possible to relieve the pain by imaging a flow of energy through the painful area.

7. Sound may be experienced as various colors of light with the eyes closed and, much less often, with the eyes open. This phenomenon is a well-known sensory crossover. It would be analogous to hear sound when light was stimulating the eyes. Stimulus of one sense appears as response in another.

8. There may be emotional discharges, such as uncontrollable laughter, crying, sometimes anger and fear, occasionally passion, sexuality, and very rarely, a sense of transcendence or a state of bliss.

9. Dreamlike images in brilliant color may occur.

10. There may be out-of-body states. There may be feelings of levitation, either with or without loss of awareness of the physical body; one may feel a sensation of being catapulted into space or to another part of the world; and one may feel one's own Beingness fusing with the group energy field and thus lose all sense of self.

11. Flashes of super-brilliant white light may be seen.

12. Three-dimensional images of Christlike or Buddhalike figures, angels, Satan, demonic creatures, loved ones who have died and members of one's family may appear.

13. Breathing patterns may slow or increase, sometimes dramatically enough to precipitate a hyperventilation syndrome. For this reaction lunch-sack-size paper bags should be available. Just place the open end of a bag lightly over the hyperventilator's nose and mouth for ten to fifteen

minutes or until the breathing pattern returns to normal. This correction should be made for anyone whose hyperventilation goes on for more than a few minutes.

14. There may be religious ecstasy states, in which people are overwhelmed with ''spiritual'' energy. They may suddenly get up off the floor and begin to sing, preach, touch people to share the ''healing'' energy, chant, speak in tongues or break into tears of ''joy.'' They are obviously not in control of their actions, and they may totally exhaust themselves unless the group leader aborts the experience.

15. Sometimes there are momentary states of confusion, disorientation and the feeling that one has gone mad.

There are myriad possible responses, but the ones I have mentioned are the most frequent. In addition, I have found an intense musical experience to be exceedingly helpful in working with individual clients, because powerful conditioning occurs when music selected by the client is played during the actual experience of energy transfer.

The client is asked to select from my record collection or to bring along a favorite piece of recorded music. While I am doing the energy-field scan and the transfer of energy through my hands, the selection is played at a comfortable volume. Later the same piece of music, played while the client is in a relaxed supine position at home, elicits a recapitulation of the body sensations experienced during the energy transfer. With a little practice, the client can learn to stimulate his or her own chakra system, and so dispense with the need for my working with the energy field. This effect engenders the feeling of self-mastery that is essential in the holistic approach to the healing art.

THE SPIRAL MEDITATION

I discussed the spiral meditation in Chapter Nine. Now I want to present an additional practice that can reinforce the exercises. While the spiral meditation is in progress, the right hand can be used to help stimulate each major chakra and all the secondary chakras except the right hand and the right elbow.

Once the attention is focused on the heart-chakra area and a physical sensation is perceived in the chest area, one images a portion of the energy of the heart chakra flowing up to the throat, over to the right shoulder and down the right arm to the hand, so that when the right palm is placed over the heart-chakra area, a circuit is established. The hand can rest lightly on the body surface or can be held several inches away from the body surface. Either hand position establishes the connection. (Left-handed people also use the right hand in this exercise.)

Note that one must move to a level of perception from which one can observe and sense both the right hand and the chakra over which the hand is located. One must not just think the energy is flowing from the heart area to the right hand and back into the heart chakra; one must *feel* the energy moving in this pattern.

The next step is to move the right hand to the solar-plexus chakra, continuing to image the heart-chakra energy moving up to the throat, over to the right shoulder, down to the right hand, on out and into the solar-plexus chakra. At the same time, one must image the heart energy flowing in a small arc toward the left and downward to the solar-plexus area within the body. The heart-chakra energy is, in other words, the only energy that stimulates itself and all other chakras in the spiral meditation, no matter whether the energy is coming from the heart area to the right hand or from the heart area in a spiral pattern to each successive chakra. I find it noteworthy that clairvoyants report a white light emanating from the center of each chakra when the awakened heart chakra is actively stimulating the other chakras.

The addition of the right hand to this exercise begins to prepare the right hand (and eventually the left hand) to sense the fields and to radiate heart-level energy to any chakra in the individual's own body or to the chakras of another person.

Note, also, that, as one leaves the throat chakra and moves on to the groin or root chakra, the line of the spiral leaves the confines of the physical body. Energy flow does not have to be maintained within the physical limits of the body. I have already stressed that the physical body is inside you: the flow of energy is *within you*, even though it is sometimes outside the physical body.

When one arrives at the point where the right elbow is being stimulated, simply image the heart energy flowing both in the spiral pattern to the right elbow and to the right shoulder, down to the right elbow — pulling the energy back from the right hand to the right elbow. When one reaches the point where the right hand is involved in the spiral pattern, simply allow the heart energy to flow in both routes to the right hand.

Since the transpersonal point is often farther above the head than the right hand can reach, image the energy radiating from the right palm to an area eighteen to twenty-four inches above the head, with the right arm and hand held over the head.

Once the opening spiral is completed, relax the right arm and hand on the right thigh and allow the meditative state to unfold. The spiral can be imaged as continuing on to infinity in its pattern.

When the meditation is over, close the spiral, beginning at the transpersonal point and reversing the pattern of the opening. Continue to image the energy as flowing from the heart chakra to the right hand and simultaneously flowing in a gradually contracting spiral pattern. Work with each chakra included in the spiral meditation and end with the heart chakra. As the last step in the exercise, withdraw the energy from the right hand back to the heart chakra.

During the closing spiral, become totally aware of each chakra and of the physical portion of the body it influences. At the end of the exercise, one should feel completely reintegrated with the body.

The spiral meditation, with the addition of the activated right hand, is the basic technique I employed in my personal meditative periods. After the first three months of daily practice, I was able to stop using the right hand and to concentrate solely on the energy flow in the spiral from the heart chakra. Since I was then working with two to four clients a day, scanning and transferring energy from both right hand and left, I no longer needed to use the right hand in the meditation.

All of the following exercises require working in pairs (dyads) or in threes (triads), changing partners at the conclusion of each exercise. A director is needed to give step-by-step instructions and to keep track of the time. The exercises are designed to give feedback to each participant so that it is certain that each person feels the energy flow occurring. The exercises are to be performed only in the sequence given here, with none omitted. They are performed only once. Most groups go through them over a one-week period, but the sequence may be completed in two days if the group's entire attention is on body-field work.

DYADIC EXERCISES

1. Following the instructions of the director, the partners of each dyad sit facing each other, either in chairs or on the floor, in positions they can hold comfortably for twenty minutes or so. In each dyad, the hands rest palm to palm, the right hand of one partner holding the left hand of the other. The eyes are closed. Each person is instructed to center the attention on his or her own heart chakra. Once the centering is complete, each participant is to imagine a chrysalis of white light surrounding the body and shielding it from any outside forces, distractions or intrusions.

(The shielding and the centering at the heart level are performed at the beginning of *all* the exercises. The basic sitting position, hand in hand, is practiced in all but one or two. It is therefore important to feel comfortable, secure and right in these basics.)

After the centering and shielding, each participant for twenty minutes does absolutely nothing but image the flow of Unconditional Love from his or her heart chakra to the heart chakra of his or her partner. For each person it is entirely a sharing, radiating action. The emphasis is on giving, and there is no concern about feeling anything coming from the partner. To love another person unconditionally even for only twenty minutes is a powerful experience, and it is not easy. The task is to be in a state of Unconditional Love, to focus through the heart chakra, and to be the radiance that one sends to the partner. In the last thirty seconds, the participants are instructed to withdraw the energy back to the heart-chakra area. As the exercise ends, the eyes are opened.

2. The second dyadic exercise precisely recapitulates the first, but after the first five minutes the participants are instructed to allow a portion of the heart-chakra energy to flow to the throat-chakra area, then to each shoulder, down each arm and to radiate from both hands to the hands of their partners. Each person is to image a fusion of the energy flow at both of his or her hands with the energy flow at both hands of the partner so that there is a ball of light around each pair of joined hands. At the same time, the radiation of energy directly from the heart chakra to the partner's heart chakra is to be maintained. The exercise continues, with energy flowing from heart to heart and from hand to hand, for an additional fifteen minutes. In the last thirty seconds of the exercise, the participants are instructed to withdraw the energy back to their own heart chakras, to disconnect hands and to open their eyes.

3. In the third exercise the partners in each dyad are arbitrarily designated #1 or #2. In the first minute they sit, center and shield. In the next four minutes they repeat Exercise 2; but the director omits the half-minute closure of Exercise 2.

After these five minutes, the #1 partners are instructed to stop transmitting any heart-chakra energy, either directly through the heart or through the hands, and to enter a completely receptive state of consciousness resting quietly in the heart-chakra area of awareness beginning the process of developing the witness — just watching or observing what is happening. The #2 partners, however, are to continue actively sending heart-chakra energy, both through the heart and through the hands. All participants observe the difference of feeling when one partner is only sending and the other is only receiving. After five minutes in this pattern, the partners reverse their roles, so that #2 is totally receptive while #1 is actively sending energy both through the heart chakra and through the hands. This pattern also continues for five minutes.

Now all participants are instructed to send energy actively through the heart chakra and through the hands. When this transmission has been established, in about thirty seconds, both partners in each dyad are instructed to let the energy from the heart chakra expand until it fills the chest, then the entire body and then the space surrounding the body; this process takes about a minute.

Now the participants are asked to do a "field embrace": each person projects his or her own field, filled with heart-chakra energy, to the field of his or her partner so that their fields overlap and interact. For five minutes, each participant tries to reach a state of fusion with his or her partner at the level of the energy field. The members of the dyads then draw their energy fields back to their own heart chakras and open their eyes. When both partners' eyes are open, the two people physically embrace each other, carefully noting the difference between the feeling of the field embrace and the feeling of the physical embrace. They then take five to ten minutes to share their experiences with each other.

4. In the fourth dyadic exercise, the partners are again numbered. For the first five minutes, they repeat the third exercise up to the conclusion of the field embrace. At this point, partner #1 is instructed to return to heart level, to withdraw all energy back to the heart area and then to establish an impenetrable shield blocking off all energy flow from partner #2. Partner #2 is instructed to attempt to break through this shield by means of energy projection only. The director of the exercise may suggest that #2 try to break through #1's shield by moving the energy around to the shielded partner's backside, or the director may suggest trying to penetrate the bottom of #1's feet. The

director intensifies the action by instructing the participants to increase their efforts either in shielding or in penetrating. When they have pushed themselves and their partners to their limits, the director instructs the #1 partner to open the shield and to notice the sensation of allowing the energy from #2 to flow inside once again while partner #2, who was trying to penetrate the shield, is instructed to notice the change in sensation when the shield opens. After a minute or two, the exercise is reversed so that partner #2 is instructed to shield and partner #1 to penetrate the shield. The director repeats the intensification process and at the peak of the interaction instructs the #1 partners to open their shields. The partners do a field embrace and end the exercise as in exercise 3. Again they take five to ten minutes to share their experience.

After the sharing time the entire group discusses the exercises thus far. It is important to go no further if any participant is having any difficulty. The most common problems are:

a. One or both partners may feel depleted or exhausted at the end of any of the exercises. This symptom indicates that they are drawing from their personal body-energy reserves. A hypothesis I am currently exploring suggests that the heart chakra (and probably other chakras) may have access to an interdimensional source of energy—that is, a source beyond anything we can conventionally imagine in the everyday reality. After participants have considered this idea, the sensation of depletion usually does not reappear in future exercises. In addition, participants are asked not to utilize the physical body's energy—either their own or their partners—but to allow an inpouring of energy from another dimension, whatever it is. As in so many other cases, it is not necessary to understand; it is necessary only to conceive the possibility.

Besides sharing energy, people can give energy to others or draw energy from others. It is called the energizer-drainer phenomenon. One person radiates energy while the other sucks it in. Beginner "radiators" may feel drained by energy "vacuum cleaners," but it is never necessary to be drained, because the consciousness of an individual can tap a source of unlimited energy that does not come from the physical plane of matter. The radiator, you must remember, is not the origin but simply the transmitter of the energy. The consciousness can not only tap this energy from the universe, but can transduce it into other kinds of energies, some of them well-known to conventional science. The human body, when awakened, is an interdimensional transducer of energy.

b. A participant may be "head-tripping" or thinking about the exercise but not allowing the *experience* of the exercise. Getting out of one's head is not easy, especially if one has been conditioned by higher education. As a part of this problem there is often the thought, "I am not doing this right," a thought that invariably and inevitably blocks experiencing anything at all. To overcome it, don't try to *do* the exercise, just *be* the exercise.

c. One may sense one's field radiating and flowing but feel nothing coming from the partner. This phenomenon usually happens to people who are great at giving but have difficulty receiving — or accepting — from others. It is based on a psychological knot of self-rejection. The more the giving is distorted with difficulty in receiving, the greater is the underlying subconscious feeling of inadequacy and unworthiness. Another good index is one's response to being given an unsolicited gift: if one's immediate psychological response is discomfort, one is clearly stuck in the psychological power dynamics of the lender and the debtor. An integrated person can accept an unsolicited gift from another without discomfort and without feeling a need to give something back.

d. One may sense energy coming from another, but not feel one's energy going to another. Again, we are talking about an aspect of self-rejection. The usual thought process is: "I can receive energy from that person, but I don't want that person to have to experience my energy."

The solution to both the c and d examples is to shift out of egocentricity, or the personality level of awareness, and move to more expanded areas where the words *unconditional sharing of one's Beingness* have meaning. At the heart level of awareness, giving and receiving are simultaneous actions, because

Love from the heart level has absolutely no strings attached. It is Unconditional, and to be in a state of Unconditional Love is to Love oneself as unconditionally as one Loves others!

5. The fifth dyadic exercise combines breath control and the spiral meditation. In it the person begins to use the breath to control the projection of energy from each chakra to the corresponding chakra of the partner.

Sitting, holding hands, centering and shielding as in exercise 1, the dyads go into a breathing pattern according to the instructions of the director.

First, the participant inhales slowly through the nose, feeling for the flow of the breath energy into the area of the heart chakra. At the peak of inspiration, the director instructs the participants to hold the breath and maintain the focus of attention on the heart chakra. After three or four seconds, each person slowly exhales through the mouth, with the tongue touching the front part of the roof of the mouth. Simultaneously, he or she images the energy from the heart chakra being projected into the partner's heart chakra.

At the end of the exhalation, he or she again inhales slowly through the nose, directing the breath energy to the heart chakra. Again he or she holds the breath at the end of the inhalation and maintains the focus on the area of the heart chakra and exhales through the mouth, directing the energy from his or her own heart chakra to the partner's heart chakra. The director has the dyads repeat this cycle enough times to establish a comfortable rhythm between the partners.

Once they have relaxed into this beginning phase of the exercise, the director instructs them to shift the process to the solar-plexus chakra on the next inhalation. His or her breath energy is directed into the solar-plexus chakra during inhalation through the nose, focused there during the holding phase, released from his or her own solar-plexus chakra and projected to the partner's solar-plexus chakra during exhalation through the mouth. After the cycle is repeated once more at the solar-plexus chakra, the dyads move on to the midchest chakra.

As the exercise continues, each person goes through the

same cycle twice at each subsequent chakra area, following the spiral pattern until the transpersonal point is reached. After breathing twice into the transpersonal point, the partners are instructed to fuse with each other's transpersonal points and to allow the breathing to return to a natural rhythm.

After ten minutes, the dyads are instructed to resume breath control and begin to reverse the spiral pattern, starting at the transpersonal point and ending at the heart chakra. In this closing of the spiral, only one breath per chakra is used. After the closure is completed at the heart chakra, the dyads resume normal breathing rhythm, do a field embrace, but instead of returning the heart-chakra energy from the field to the heart chakra, the energy fields are to remain expanded as each partner goes into a physical embrace, noting the additional quality of a simultaneous physical and field embrace.

6. The sixth dyadic exercise is the first to emphasize the projection of the heart-chakra energy through the opened eyes. It begins, like the second exercise, by allowing several minutes for the dyads to achieve hand and heart connections. The participants are then instructed to image a flow of part of the heart-chakra energy upward through (but not out of) the midchest and the throat chakras to the area behind the eyes.

When the energy reaches the areas of the eyes, the participants open their eyes and each person projects the ascending heart energy through the eyes to the partner's eyes. If one partner finds that the other partner's eyes are not yet open, the energy must be held at the eyes until the partner's eyes are opened. Blinking of the eyes is permissible. At this point, each participant should be aware of the heart-chakra energy in three simultaneous patterns. The first, heart chakra to heart chakra; the second, from hands to hands; the third, from eyes to eyes.

When the participants sense the energy release through the eyes, they close them and image the energy as returning back down to the heart chakra. This exercise is repeated ten times and ends as does exercise 5.

7. The seventh dyadic exercise is the first of the exercises to incorporate the voice. Silence has been maintained during the previous exercises. This exercise begins as does exercise 6, but the energy is imaged as rising only to the throat chakra. As the energy reaches that point, each participant is to vocalize the sound of the heart-chakra energy, finding a single tone to sing or to hum to harmonize with the tone from his or her partner. The eyes remain closed. After about a minute of vocalizing, the participants are instructed to become silent and return the energy back to the heart chakra, as in exercise 6. Again the exercise is repeated ten times and ends as does exercise 5.

8. The eighth dyadic exercise combines exercises 6 and 7. As each participant raises the energy from the heart chakra to the throat chakra, he or she vocalizes a single note and simultaneously raises a portion of the heart-chakra energy to the eyes. Then the eyes are opened so that the partners are simultaneously in vocal contact, eye contact, hand contact and heart-chakra contact. After about a minute, the eyes are closed and the energy withdrawn to the throat. Vocalization ends as the energy is withdrawn back to the heart chakra. This exercise is repeated three times and ends as does exercise 5.

9. The ninth dyadic exercise is a repetition of the fifth exercise, except that the partners are back to back, so that the awareness of the posterior fields is developed. Each participant's hands are resting on his or her own thighs. Just before the end of the exercise, each person is instructed to focus a portion of the heart-chakra energy at the throat chakra and, while vocalizing a single tone, to feel the sound from the partner vibrating the back of the chest area. At the conclusion, still back to back, the partners engage in a field embrace. The closing is as in exercise 1.

10. The tenth dyadic exercise explores the disintegration of the sense of touch. *The key to the breakdown of any of the five*

outer senses is fixation of that sense. In the case of touch, the partners are instructed to hold each other's hands without moving them. Any movement of the hands will break the state of concentration.

The exercise begins exactly as does exercise 1. After ten to fifteen seconds, the participants are instructed to place their entire attention into their hands. Each partner is to be totally receptive, aware of only the information coming from the hands of his or her partner. From this single connection they are to sense for temperature, pulsation, texture, sound, color and vibration. After five minutes, they are instructed to forget they are holding each other's hands and to allow spontaneous images to appear in the minds about the "object" they are touching. The task, in other words, is to detach from the knowledge that hands are being held, to allow the self to feel that something else is being held and to allow that something else to be imaged in the mind. Rarely will both partners image the same "object." This part of the exercise takes fifteen minutes.

At the end of this time, the participants are instructed to hold the left hand passive and slowly move the fingers of the right hand. This action will immediately return the focus of the participants' awareness to the sense of touch. Participants must now shift their awareness to a perspective where they are aware of receiving stimuli *simultaneously* through the passive left hand and through the active right hand. No oscillation of awareness from one hand to the other hand is allowed. The active right hand is to explore light touch, pressure and rhythm, feeling every physical aspect of the partner's passive left hand. In both partners, the left hand is passive and the right hand actively exploring, while the focus of awareness is centered simultaneously on both hands and on both activities.

After several minutes, the partners are instructed to make their right hands passive and their left hands active and to repeat the action as before. Finally, both hands of both partners are activated, each partner maintaining simultaneous awareness of both the activity and the sensory input from both hands. The exercise ends as does exercise 3.

11. The eleventh dyadic exercise explores the telepathic potential of the participants. As in exercise 3, the partners are designated #1 or #2 and begin with the usual centering and shielding.

Partner #1 is instructed to select a pure feeling tone—such as joy, anger, inspiration, Love, sexuality, excitement—and allow it to develop fully. At the same time, he or she locates the chakra in the body that most closely relates to the feeling tone and projects the feeling tone through that chakra to the corresponding chakra of partner #2.

After several minutes, partner #2 describes what he or she is feeling while partner #1, in silence, maintains the feeling tone that he or she has been projecting.

Partner #1 then describes the chakra and the feeling tone that he or she transmitted. Both partners are then instructed to recenter, as at the beginning of the exercise.

Partner #2 is again receptive, while partner #1 selects a feeling tone and a chakra—either different or the same as before—and again projects to partner #2. After several minutes, partner #2 is asked to describe what was felt and where, and then partner #1 describes what he or she was transmitting.

After the entire process has been repeated three times, the situation is reversed so that partner #1 becomes receptive and partner #2 the selector and transmitter. Again the exercise is repeated three times.

The participants are then instructed to recenter. Partner #2 is now to become receptive while partner #1 is to connect with partner #2, heart chakra to heart chakra, and to image a geometric form and project it through his or her forehead chakra to the forehead chakra of partner #2. At the same time, partner #1 is to activate the throat chakra and silently project the name of the geometric form from his or her throat chakra to the throat chakra of partner #2.

At this point, partner #1 should be simultaneously (a) connecting his or her heart chakra with the heart chakra of partner #2; (b) silently vocalizing the name of the geometric form and projecting the word from the throat chakra to the throat chakra of partner #2; and (c) projecting the image of the geometric form from his or her forehead chakra to the forehead chakra of partner #2.

After five minutes, partner #2 is asked to report what geometric form was received. This segment of the exercise is now repeated, with partner #1 selecting either another geometric form or the same one.

After the partners have compared what was transmitted with what was received, they reverse their roles so that partner #1 becomes the receiver and partner #2 the transmitter. The same procedure is followed by partner #2—and again the segment is repeated. The exercise ends as does exercise 5.

As I have said elsewhere in this book, in telepathy you do not actually send or transmit anything to another person as a beam or wave through space. You impress that portion of your personal holographic negative where the person with whom you wish to communicate is located. All holographic negatives in every human being are simultaneously impressed. The trick in telepathy is for the specific individual represented in your hologram to be sensitive enough to realize that the portion of his or her hologram representing you is communicating with him or her!

12. The twelfth dyadic exercise explores the disintegration of the sense of sight. It is a modification of the Trespasso exercises used by the Tibetans, Sufis and certain Western esoteric schools. It is the most uncomfortable of the exercises to perform, because it requires the participants to stare without blinking for twenty-five to thirty minutes. The staring is necessary—even the slightest movement of the eye will cause the phenomenon which develops in this exercise to cease abruptly.

It is called the Trespasso exercise because one trespasses within the outer barrier of a person when one peers into his or her eyes—especially the left eye, since it is considered the portal to the soul. This thought follows old tradition, and, as one experiences the eye exercises over a period of months or years, there is much to suggest that it is valid.

This exercise is best conducted in the evening, because the lighting in the room should be subdued without being actually dark. Then, at the conclusion of the eye exercises—which entail three periods of staring, each twenty-five to thirty minutes long—the participants can rest their eyes overnight. A hot moist towel over the eyes at bedtime is enough to ease any discomfort. In my experiences with over 500 people there has never been any reported injury to the eye created by this exercise.

People who wear glasses or contact lenses are to remove them before the exercise. Prolonged staring while wearing contact lenses can be injurious to the eyes. Glasses tend to create a psychological buffer between the partners. The partners are to seat themselves comfortably facing each other and as close to each other as possible. Each participant rests the hands on his or her own thighs. At the beginning, the eyes are kept closed while the director gives the instructions.

While the participants are centering with their eyes closed, the director instructs them to pretend they have purchased a ticket to a show. No matter what a participant sees during the staring process, each is only to witness the visual changes, without reacting to what he or she sees. The participants are further instructed to maintain the focus of the eyes on a single point and not to move either the head or the body. Each person must remain absolutely motionless. If the eyes tear, the participant is to allow the tears, without bringing the hands up to the face. Each participant is to allow the eyelids to drop slightly and to relax into the staring process. Each participant is again instructed to center and to shield and is reminded not to react to anything he or she sees. They are told that after they open their eyes, they are to focus on the pupil of the left eye of their partners. Only after these instructions are given are the eyes opened.

The director leaves the room and returns in twenty-five minutes. The participants are then instructed to close their eyes and to pay particular attention to the afterimages they see. Facial tissue is available. The partners in each dyad share their experience for fifteen minutes.

The second twenty-five minute segment is the same as the first except that each participant focuses his or her eyes on the root of the partner's nose, between the eyebrows.

In the third twenty-five minute segment, the participants may elect to stare either at the partner's left pupil or at the bridge of the nose. Ten minutes into the exercise, they try to see whether they can make anything they choose appear as images in their minds. Fifteen minutes into the exercise, they are asked to maintain the focal point of their eyes but simultaneously to pay attention only to the light surrounding the partner's head. Twenty minutes into the exercise, the participants are asked to remain fixed on the original point of focus and to change the sex of the partner's face. Twenty-five minutes into the exercise, they are asked to see whether they can allow images of a past life of the partner to emerge into their awareness.

At the end of thirty minutes, the partners close their eyes and share their experiences for twenty minutes. Then there is a group sharing, in which it is important to concentrate on the significance of the exercise in breaking down the usual experiences of vision.

These eye exercises are powerful experiences. The director must be ready to handle the emotional content that may arise both during and after the exercises.

Finally, each person is to perform the Trespasso exercise alone, using a mirror. Most people will want to wait until their eyes are rested before proceeding any further.

To avoid influencing the reader, I am not going to share the experiences that people have during this exercise. Many esoteric schools require aspirants to perform the exercise with a mirror for half an hour, twice daily, for indefinite periods of time. It is extremely valuable in learning to comprehend how the mind can operate, especially in distorting external reality.

The eye exercises are the beginning steps into clairvoyant vision, crystal-ball work, tea-leaf reading and higher techniques of Tarot-card reading, all of which tap dimensions of awareness beyond the outer mind.

13. The thirteenth dyadic exercise begins the process of energy transfer through either hand to a partner, both with and without physical contact.

The initial positioning of the dyads is as in exercise 1. The partners are designated #1 and #2. The eyes remain closed as the participants center and shield. Partner #2, in a totally receptive state of consciousness, is to focus attention on the hands. Partner #1 is to direct energy from the heart chakra through either the right hand or the left hand to partner #2. Partner #2, not knowing which hand partner #1 is using, attempts to distinguish the hand only by the energy flow that he or she feels. Partner #1 is to "turn off" any energy flow from the hand that is not radiating the heart-chakra energy. Since the hands are in contact, it is important to avoid giving partner #2 such clues as a slight motion of the hand that is sending the energy, slight increases of pressure and so on. After several minutes, partner #2 is asked to squeeze the hand that is radiating the energy flow. Both partners are to remain silent.

Partner #1 is then instructed to select either the same hand or the other hand to repeat the process. Again, after several minutes, partner #2 is to squeeze the hand that is transmitting the energy. This sequence is repeated for a total of five times before the roles are reversed, and partner #1 becomes totally receptive, while partner #2 activates either the right hand or the left hand with heart-chakra energy. Again, partner #2 has five opportunities to select either hand to activate, and partner #1 has five opportunities to determine which hand partner #2 has activated.

Partner #1 is now asked to position his or her hands, palm-side down, approximately three inches above the hands of partner #2. Partner #2 is asked to become totally receptive, with the hands held palm-side up and resting on the thighs. Partner #1 is instructed to activate one hand and radiate heart-chakra energy from that hand to the hand of partner #2. Partner #1 must image the energy flow moving through the space between the radiating hand and the receiving hand of partner

#2, and he or she is reminded to "turn off" the energy in the unactivated hand. After several minutes, partner #2 raises the hand that is receiving the energy flow and lightly touches the partner's hand that was receiving. Both partners' eyes remain closed. This sequence is repeated for a total of five times, with one further variation: partner #1 can activate the right hand, the left hand or both hands, and partner #2 is aware of this possibility.

Then the roles are reversed, and partner #1 rests his or her hands on the thighs, palm side up, while partner #2 holds his or her hands about three inches above, palm side down. The entire sequence is repeated for a total of five times, as in the previous segment.

Then the roles are reversed again. The same procedure is followed, but this time partner #1 holds his or her hands six to eight inches above the hands of partner #2. The sequence is repeated as before, allowing each partner five opportunities to transmit and to receive energy flow.

In the final sequence, the partners' hands are twelve to eighteen inches apart. At this distance, when it is time for the receiver to inform the sender, it may be necessary for the receiver to open his or her eyes to see where the partner's hand is in order to be able to touch it. Again, each partner has five opportunities to send and to receive. The closing is as in exercise 5.

The dyadic exercises are now concluded. If a person in the last exercise could not determine which hand the partner was activating, he or she is to continue with the exercise until it is mastered.

Most participants in the ranch Conferences have little difficulty with the last dyadic exercise. In fact, most find it easier to send and receive energy at a distance than to do it when the hands are in physical contact. It never ceases to amaze me how fast participants can learn to do these energy exercises. Perhaps it is because by the time they are attempting this last exercise, I have already demonstrated to each of them my own ability to pass energy in this manner. I suspect this demonstration catalyzes their ability. When most participants can perform the thirteenth exercise with few errors, the series of triadic exercises (three people participating) can commence.

TRIADIC EXERCISES

The triadic exercises resemble the dyadic exercises but are complicated by the addition of the third person.

1. In the first triadic exercise, the three people are instructed to arrange themselves in a triangular pattern, facing inward. They can sit on the floor or in chairs. Each individual holds the hand of the partner on either side and rests the hands on the knees, which are touching a partner's knee on each side. All participants center and shield. The eyes are closed during the exercise.

After about a minute to establish a base, the participants are instructed to spend twenty minutes exploring the new configuration, feeling out the differences between dyadic relationship and triadic relationships. Each person must make adjustments for the differences between the partners on either side.

Each person is now holding one hand of each of two individuals, instead of both hands of one individual, as in the dyadic exercises. Quantitative and qualitative differences between the hands of the partners on each side can be determined — differences of temperature, moisture, pulsation and vibration. The exercise is performed in silence and without motion.

At the end of twenty minutes, the members of each triad are to center at heart level and expand the heart-chakra energy until each individual's field is radiating heart-chakra energy; then, as a unit, they are to perform a field embrace. After several minutes, they are instructed to return the energy to their heart chakras, open their eyes and, as a unit, do a physical embrace. Then they share their experiences for ten minutes.

2. The second triadic exercise explores the potential of the members of the triad to fuse as a unit. After beginning as in the first triadic exercise, each participant is to image a beam of

energy radiating from the heart chakra and extending to the center of the triangle. After approximately one minute, all members of the triad are asked to allow the focus of awareness to leave the confines of the physical body and become the center of the triangle. When the awareness is at the center of the triangle, each participant—without opening the eyes—is to observe his or her body as it sits forming one side of the triangle. After a participant, eyes closed, can see a detailed image of his or her own body from the perspective of the center of the triangle, he or she is to view the two other partners in the triad in a similar fashion from the same central point of view. Five minutes is allotted for this segment.

The members of each triad are then to fuse their awareness at the center of their triangle and to lose all sense of their individual selves. Five minutes is alloted to this segment.

Now the participants are instructed to allow this fused state of consciousness to expand and fill first the room, then the building, the geographic area and so on and on, to the entire planet and, finally, on out through the solar system to infinity. Five minutes is alloted for this segment.

The participants then are instructed gradually to contract their fused awareness back through the solar system, the planet Earth, a smaller and smaller geographic area, to the building and the room, until finally they come to their fusion of awareness at their own triangle. The exercise concludes as does the first triadic exercise, with the field embrace and the triangular physical embrace. The members of each triad spend whatever time they need to share this experience.

3. The third triadic exercise explores both the problem of threes and the resolution of threes. The problem—the famous and classic "eternal triangle"—is to be resolved through the exercise of the trinity. The exercise begins like triadic exercise 1. After the participants are centered and shielded, they are instructed to explore the triangle. Then each of them is to begin—using no means other than the expression of energy flow through a hand—to make a connection with *just one* of the

other two members of the triangle. As in previous exercises, each participant must take care to give no signal by hand pressure or movement and to use energy flow alone.

For convenience in this discussion, I will name the triad members as A, B, and C, but they need not be designated in practice.

If A, after a reasonable period of time, feels no return of energy flow from B (the one he or she is trying to contact), he or she can assume that B is trying to connect with C. The energy of the unactivated hand is to be deliberately turned off during the attempt to make a contact; but if A, trying to contact B, feels energy coming to the unactivated hand from C, he or she is to stop trying to contact B and instead form a connection with C, that is, he or she is to turn off the hand touching B and turn on the hand touching C.

According to these instructions, only two of the three members of each triad can be in connection. The third person has been unable to make a connection and is, in old game terms, "out." This third person must figure out how to be in the triangle when he or she cannot be a part of the dyad formed by the other two. He or she must turn off the energy flow from both hands and still be a part of the interaction between the other two.

The director instructs the participants to intensify their activity, then says that the members who are connected are to squeeze the hand that is in connection. If communication were perfect, two hands of the six in the triad would squeeze each other; but this communication, like most others, is not always perfect: A may feel connection with B, while B does not feel connection with A. It is possible for all three people in the triad to squeeze a hand (in which case none of the squeezed hands squeezes back), and it is fairly common for each of the three to feel that the other two made contact, so that each thinks that he or she is out; then no one in the triad squeezes any hand.

After going through the procedure once, the participants recenter and repeat the process, trying new connections. The sequence is repeated for a total of five times, and the exercise ends as does triadic exercise 1.

4. The fourth triadic exercise recapitulates triadic exercise 3, except that the hands of the members of the triangle are held apart three, six and twelve inches in successive attempts to make connection with a partner by means of energy flow alone. It makes no difference whose hand is above or below, as long as the hands are positioned palm toward palm. When it is time to indicate the connection made in the triangle, the two who are in energy connection touch each other's hands. The sequence is repeated for a total of five times and ends as does triadic exercise 1.

5. The fifth triadic exercise explores vocalization and eye contact. This exercise begins, as does triadic exercise 1, with centering, shielding, closed eyes and silence. After a few minutes, each participant is instructed to allow a portion of the heart-chakra energy to flow to the throat chakra and each participant vocalizes a tone that represents the energy of the triad. When all three are vocalizing a tone (or tones — not necessarily the same one), they are to explore sound in their triad, pitching their voices to various tones. This experience continues for ten minutes. The eyes remain closed.

The director then instructs the participants to recenter at the heart chakra. After thirty to forty seconds, they are instructed to raise the heart-chakra energy to the area behind their eyes. When the energy from the heart chakra reaches the eye area, each participant opens the eyes and makes eye contact with *one* of the other two people in the triad. Again, one member will find no one with whom to make an eye connection and will have to figure out how to handle having the eyes open without being in eye contact with a partner. The two members of the dyad within the triad are to image heart-chakra energy flowing through their eyes while they simultaneously radiate heart-chakra energy through their connecting hands and through heart-chakra fields to each other.

The participants are now told that they will be repeating this process with less and less time in each repetition in succession, to make a new connection with the eyes, hands and heart-chakra fields in the dyads within the triads. They are now instructed to break eye contact and, using the eyes to make a connection with a partner, to form a new dyad within the triad. The odd person out must keep the eyes open, even though he or she establishes no eye contact. (Blinking the eyes is permissible.) As the new dyad is formed, its two members are instructed to intensify their hand and eye contact.

The participants are then instructed to break the eye contact and to form another new dyad within the triad, again with eye contact. Six seconds are allotted for this action.

The members are again asked to break eye contact and form a new dyad, and four seconds are allotted.

With the director using the words "Break, new dyad" to call for a change on the next and subsequent dyad formations, only two seconds are allotted for each cycle. The participants are reminded that they must make contact with the eyes, the hands and the heart chakra each time they enter a dyadic relationship. When the participants show the effects of the stress of this exercise, the director instructs them to do a triangular physical embrace and thus end the exercise.

In each of these triadic exercises where dyads are formed, the odd person should be able to move to a state where his or her consciousness sees the dyad fused into a single unit — and then the odd person fuses with it. The odd person, therefore, experiences unity in diversity. This is the resolution of the eternal triangle — neither to be excluded nor to win one of the partners out of the dyad but to see the dyad as a unit and to fuse with it.

The second point to be emphasized is that the participants must be able to project heart-chakra energy to another person through the hands, the voice and the eyes in less than a second. The sharing of Unconditional Love is what this training is all about. When one has mastered the energy flow of the heart chakra, Unconditional Love flows instantly to another. It does not matter whether the energy is returned. It is a universal energy to be shared. It is inexhaustible!

Too many individuals experience what I call "canteen

consciousness.'' They get high on Unconditional Love in meditation, at religious services or in the presence of people expressing Unconditional Love; but within a few hours or a few days, as they go back into the "normal" human perspective, they run out of the energy. They have not yet learned how to tap this energy flow instantly and moment by moment. The task is not easy, because more than 99 percent of humanity expresses energies other than Unconditional Love, and the pull of the collective human field is often overwhelming. In this transitional period in human development, it is difficult enough just to maintain sporadic contact with the heart level of awareness. The sharing of Unconditional Love must be a lifelong practice.

People who have completed all these exercises are ready to sense the human energy fields at a distance from the body, to transfer heart-chakra energy to another human being through their hands, and to balance the chakra system of the person with whom they are interacting. As a byproduct of this work, they may be able to relieve pain and to alter the course of disease.

What counts is not the intensity of the energy being emitted, but its quality. It is easy to transfer sexual energy, emotional energy and mental energy, and all these energies can affect another individual in both positive and negative ways. Heart-chakra energy invariably augments all souls: it cannot be other than positive.

Don't get lost in the *power* of the energy. The ego can easily swell, but this practice must not become an ego trip. It is not your energy, anyway: it is Ours. You are simply allowing it to pass into and through you, sharing it with the manifest plane. When you express Unconditional Love, you are acting as a transducer for an energy not of this world.

HAND SCANNING

This section is a detailed description of how to use the hands to detect the energy fields emanating from the human body. The practice is called "hand scanning."

In a previous chapter, I discussed the location of the

anterior fields and how they may feel to different individuals. I want to emphasize again that the energy fields are not in a frequency range known to most modern scientists. The energy fields are there, and the human body, as an instrument, can detect them. In most instances, the individual must be trained to detect the energy fields. The mere fact that the ordinary human awareness does not feel or see the fields does not disprove their presence!

As I also said before, the body-energy fields are capable of stimulating a number of different sensory systems in the hands — heat receptors, cold receptors, vibratory receptors, pressure receptors, light-touch receptors and pain receptors. In different individuals different sensory modalities predominate as the primary sensing systems for body energy, but the vast majority of people sense the fields as a subtle warmth or a subtle coldness. Only a few individuals will be able to detect the fields with more than one sensory modality. A rare individual will begin to see fragments of the fields. Even though many people sense the energy as heat or cold, it is definitely known that the energy is not a temperature phenomenon.

During the hand-scanning phase of the body-energy work, the consciousness of the scanner must become totally receptive and his or her awareness must be centered entirely in the hand or hands. The witness state of consciousness is activated. One must be careful not to project what one thinks should be there into the space surrounding the person to be scanned. Instead, the task is to explore the space surrounding the person to be scanned in order to find out what is actually there.

The hand that is acting as the detector is relaxed. The fingers should be slightly apart and may be slightly bent, as in a classical ballet pose. A rigid flat hand, with the fingers held tightly together, is not nearly so effective a detector.

Since in some individuals the forearm is more sensitive than the hand in detecting body-energy fields, the skin surface from the hand to the elbow should be exposed; long sleeves should be rolled up.

Individuals who are just beginning to learn the hand-scanning technique are to explore the fields first with the right hand, then with the left hand. Rarely is a beginner able to detect the fields equally well with both hands. Left-handed persons usually find the left hand more sensitive. Eventually, the sensitivity of both hands will be developed.

The speed at which the hand moves in space is critical. Too fast a motion will not allow the mind enough time to register the sensory input, because there is always a slight lag between the time the stimulus strikes the receptor and the time the stimulus reaches the brain. By the time one becomes aware of the sensation, the hand has always passed the place where the energy struck it. One soon learns to compensate for this divergence.

If, at the other extreme, the hand moves too slowly across the body, the scanner will often feel his or her own hand energy being reflected back from the body surface. In this case, every portion of the area over the body surface will feel the same to the scanner. An effective, practical speed is usually about a foot every two seconds.

In addition, beginners frequently have the sensation that the scanning hand is becoming "overcharged." It begins to tingle or to pulsate, sometimes with an aching sensation or with pain. The sensation blocks any other awareness of incoming stimuli. Resting the hand or flicking the fingers will usually alleviate the sensation. Patting the hand on one's own thigh often helps. Using the other hand may also alleviate the problem.

Trying to feel the fields tends to block sensory awareness. The sensation of the body energies must be *allowed* to enter the awareness. The awareness of the scanner must become attuned to a level where the energy can be felt. There is a comparable situation in medical school when students are taught to detect certain heart murmurs; first they must learn where to center their hearing awareness, because their ordinary hearing mechanism simply does not listen in the ranges where these murmurs can be heard. The same is true with the subtle sense of touch, at least at the beginning stages.

I recommend beginning approximately eight to twelve inches away from the body surface, with the person to be scanned lying face up on a table at the height of the scanner's groin. The table may be covered with a mattress, but a thinner, firmer pad is preferable. Working on the floor is fine, except that it may be uncomfortable for the scanner, particularly when scanning areas on the subject's left side, the opposite side from where the scanner is positioned. Wooden tables are preferable to metal tables, because of the intensity of the energy field radiating from metallic objects.

Gold, silver, semiprecious and precious stones, even the more common minerals, have very strong fields radiating from them. Amulets in ancient times were not for decoration, nor was their effect based on superstition. The fields radiating from certain stones are capable of influencing the body's energy fields. When charged with energy from the hands, crystals are especially powerful, as are many other stones used in jewelry. Because of the residual energy in these kinds of matter, persons to be scanned should remove all jewelry, including watches and large rings. Men should remove large belt buckles. However, there is no need to disrobe. (The scanner may or may not want to remove personal jewelry.)

The subject to be scanned is instructed to enter a quiet, relaxed state of consciousness. The subject's feet should be at least twelve inches apart and the hands resting comfortably at the sides. The subject should feel free to move arms or legs if they become uncomfortable, or to cough, sneeze or scratch if necessary. Talking during scanning is to be strongly discouraged.

The scanner first approaches the right side of the subject. The scanner's right hand feels for the pulse at the subject's right wrist. If you do not know how to feel for the pulse at the wrist, ask a nurse or a physician to teach you. I prefer the three-fingered method of pulse taking, similar to the technique used in oriental acupuncture. For the beginning scanner, it is enough to be able to feel the pulsation of the wrist artery and use it to attune one's consciousness to that of the subject.

While the scanner is feeling the pulse, he or she shifts the awareness to the heart-chakra level and performs the process of centering and shielding. Moving into a totally receptive state, the scanner then focuses the attention entirely in the scanning hand.

For the newcomer to body-energy work, I recommend beginning by scanning over the chest and the upper and lower abdominal areas, where the energy fields are usually the strongest and thus easiest to detect. It is helpful to begin the scan off to one side of the subject's body, and to work back and forth both over the surface of the body, and beyond the edge of the surface of the body, to give the necessary contrast to the scanning hand; the motion in this case is away from the body and over the body area, away from the body and over the body. After one becomes familiar with the feeling of the body-energy fields and can easily detect them, one no longer needs this strong contrast and so can work exclusively over the body.

It is through trial and error that one detects the first energy field. I recommend that the eyes be closed in order to avoid diverting the concentration and to hold it entirely in the hands. While some people sense the fields immediately, others may feel the first sensations only vaguely. The key to the method is to work in contrasting areas.

The fields are not felt while the hand is held over them but as the hand moves through them. This principle is fundamental. During a scan, the hand must be in constant motion. It must pass in and out of the fields. If it remains in a field, little will be felt. The task is to slice through the radiating field at different levels and thus conceive what the field's configuration must be. Its diameter and the angle of projection can be detected only by constantly moving the sensing hand in and out of the field at various levels from the body surface. Do not conclude that the field is radiating from directly below the hand. One must make a series of explorations of the field, before any conclusion as to its source can be made.

Once a field is encountered, one determines the distance of its projection, its diameter at various levels and its angle from the surface of the body. The distance to which the field seems to radiate from the body surface is initially a function of the sensitivity of the scanner. (I find the fields two to three times farther from the body than the beginner does.) At the beginning, however, it is enough just to detect the fields from each of the chakra areas included in the spiral meditation. These major fields—especially those from the groin to the top of the head—are the ones most easily detected. As part of this first scan, one assesses the differences in intensity of the fields from each of the chakras.

Several discriminations are difficult. The throat chakra is often confused with the warmth from the subject's breath. To avoid this confusion, ask the subject to hold his or her breath while you check for the throat chakra. To facilitate the detection of the throat chakra, it may also be necessary to elevate the chin so that the scanning hand is not in line with either mouth or nostrils.

The throat, midchest, heart and solar-plexus chakras are close together, but their fields are always discrete: particular care must be taken to separate them in the scan. The lower-abdomen and groin chakras are often confused because they, too, are close together. But they, too, are always discrete, and one's sensitivity must be heightened to distinguish them.

Concentrating on only the fields included in the spiral meditation will save much time and energy. There are more than forty normal, discrete fields radiating from the body surfaces, front, back and side. Most are so subtle that great sensitivity is necessary to detect them. Occasionally, strong energy fields are felt over the breast areas of females, and over the umbilical area of both men and women. If you feel them, fine; otherwise, concentrate on the spiral-meditation fields.

When learning to hand scan, it is advantageous to work with a group of people, because different subjects will show different intensities in the various energy fields. Exploring the energy fields of a person whose energies are very subtle, one might conclude that the fields are not there or that one is incapable of sensing them, but then the next person's strong, easily detected energy fields can provide reassurance that one is indeed able to sense fields.

On completing the exploration of the fields that project from the front of the body, ask the partner to turn over, so that the posterior fields can be detected. Since I have not commented on where these fields are located, each scanner has the opportunity to discover them without knowing their locations ahead of time. (See Fig. 10.20, pg. 276. Please refrain from studying the illustration until after having the opportunity to feel the posterior field.)

While the subject is lying face down, scan under the table, if it is physically possible, and examine the fields that you explored while the subject was lying face up. The fields penetrate through anything. If you remove the block in your mind that considers the table an obstruction to the energy fields, you will find that they are easy to detect. But be sure that your scanning hand is at least six inches away from the lower surface of the table, so that you won't feel the energy from your own hand reflected back from it. At this juncture scan both above and below the table simultaneously (bimanual scanning), to ascertain whether the anterior and posterior field are connected.

As a final exercise, ask the subject to turn over again to expose the front side. Have the subject raise one or the other of his or her hands, so that the forearm and hand are perpendicular to the table, with the upper arm resting on the table. Then completely scan the raised open hand, checking the back side, the palm and the fingertips at a distance of approximately six inches. Then ask the subject to turn the hand on — as in the dyadic and triadic exercises — and scan the hand fields again, noting the increase of intensity and where the intensity seems greatest. Ask the subject to turn the hand off and then recheck the fields. If you want an additional test of your ability to detect energy fields, ask the subject to turn the hand on and off at will, without your knowledge, and then indicate to the subject when you think the hand is activated and when it is not.

If you sense little in your initial exploration of body-energy fields, try again in twenty-four hours. Often, apprehension about feeling the fields subsides and the next day's exploration is much more satisfactory. Since less than 1 percent of people are totally unable to detect the fields, the odds are greatly in your favor.

The ability to detect the fields is critical in the next phase of the body-energy work, the transfer of energy to a subject. One cannot tell where to transmit the energy, nor how much to transmit, without being able to sense the fields. Practice the scanning technique until most, if not all, of the chakras of the spiral meditation can be felt.

THE TRANSFER OF BODY ENERGY

Performing the energy-transfer technique requires a high degree of concentration. Both the person to whom the energy is being transferred (the subject) and the person transferring energy (the operator) become vulnerable to forces of which most human beings are totally unaware. One must be constantly aware of the quality and the intensity of energy being transferred, because it is all too easy to disrupt the functioning of a chakra temporarily.

To minimize the complications that may occur, the subject is asked to act as a biofeedback instrument, constantly monitoring the energy flowing into the body and reporting to the operator whether the energy is too little, too intense or just right. If the energy flow feels good, no matter what the intensity, no deleterious effects will manifest.

Thus, the persons receiving energy in this final exercise are totally responsible for what happens to them. The operator is responsible for the quality and the intensity of the energy and for regulating its flow according to the instructions of the subject. There must be mutual trust between operator and subject.

The exercise may take sixty to ninety minutes to complete. In a group situation, the director can pace the various sequences, suggesting when each phase should be nearing completion, but ample time is always to be allotted for each phase. For this exercise in particular, the director must be both sensitive and experienced.

During the actual energy-transfer portion of this exercise, the operator must not only activate the hand that will transfer the heart-chakra energy, but also, simultaneously, enter a sensing state to feel the flow of energy and the response of the chakra over which the hand is being held. During scanning, the hand is always in motion; during transfer, it is held motionless over each chakra in turn.

The intensity of energy radiating from the hand can be controlled by three methods. One way is to image a regulator valve or rheostat that allows more or less energy to flow through it, depending upon the flow of energy you desire. If this method doesn't work, then you can vary the distance between the radiating hand and the body surface at the chakra. Working farther away from the body will decrease the intensity felt by the subject, and working closer to the body surface will increase it. Sometimes it is necessary to work two or three feet away from the body surface, and at others it will be necessary to rest the hand lightly upon the clothing; the distances vary not only from operator to operator but also from subject to subject and chakra to chakra in the same subject. The third method is for the operator to utilize breathing ''into'' the heart and hand areas as in dyadic exercise 5.

Before commencing the exercise, the partners should work out nonverbal cues for the subject to tell the operator when and in which direction to modulate the energy flow. In one convenient set of signals, the subject raises one finger to indicate too little energy flow and thus ask for more; two fingers to indicate that the flow of energy is just right; and three fingers to indicate too much energy and to ask for less. Because the operator is ordinarily standing at the subject's right side, signals given by the subject's right hand would be out of the operator's normal range of vision; if subject and operator are in the usual positions, the signals are best given by both hands of the subject simultaneously. The cues should be exaggerated so that they cannot be misunderstood, and the subject should continuously reflect the feeling of the energy flow, moment by moment: the subject should always be giving one signal or another. Since the operator frequently works with eyes closed, the subject may have to snap his or her fingers or touch the working partner to signal that a change is indicated. The subject must not go off into a dream world while the exercise is in process.

Before starting the exercise, it is also desirable for the subject to tell the operator the exact location of any pain or discomfort in the body, so that the operator knows ahead of time where to concentrate during this segment of the exercise.

To avoid breaking the operator's concentration, the subject must not speak. Even whispering is not permitted. The only sounds that should be heard are occasional snaps of the fingers to remind the operator to look at the finger cues. A background of serene music may be used to help set the ambience.

There are eight segments to the exercise:
1. Centering, attuning and shielding
2. Hand scanning
3. Opening spiral-chakra work with energy transfer
4. Connection of chakras with energy transfer
5. Relief of pain or discomfort and intuitive work
6. Final hand scanning with last-minute balancing
7. Closing spiral-chakra work
8. Release

The centering of one's awareness at heart level should have been mastered during the earlier exercises. It is essential, because it determines the quality of the energy that will be transmitted. As in the initial hand-scanning exercise, the centering, shielding and attunement to the subject occur while the pulse is being taken, and the rhythm of the pulse intensifies the connection between the partners.

The hand-scanning segment is the same as in the previous exercise except that only the fields radiating from the front of the partner on the table are examined. I recommend starting from the transpersonal point, if it can be felt, or from the crown chakra and slowly scanning down to the feet, checking the elbows and hands during the scanning of the chest and abdominal areas. The task in this scan is to note the relative intensity of each chakra in order to determine which chakras need more or less energy during the later transferring process. During this scan, the operator's hand must be kept in constant motion. The operator's state of consciousness is receptive, the awareness focused in the hand detecting the fields. The subject may feel some energy coming from the hand of the operator. Unless it causes discomfort, there is no need to signal the operator during this segment. It is during the next three segments that the feedback is required from the partner on the table.

When the scanning is completed, the operator should return to the chest area to begin the stimulation of each chakra in the pattern used in the spiral meditation, commencing at the heart chakra and going eventually to the transpersonal point. The operator must now change levels of awareness, activate the heart-chakra energy and image it flowing to the shoulder and to the hand that is used for transferring the energy. I recommend having the hand approximately six inches away from the body surface, beginning at low intensity and allowing the subject to guide the increase in intensity with the finger cues. The operator will feel a "connection" with the chakra in anything from thirty seconds to several minutes. *Image* the energy flowing into the partner's body at the heart-chakra area at the same time that you *feel* the energy flowing to the partner. The task during this segment is not to balance the chakras, but to stimulate them with the heart-chakra energy from the operator. Approximately two minutes should be spent at each chakra area. Unconditional Love is the state of consciousness during transfer work.

After completing the stimulation of the forehead chakra in the spiral pattern, one would ordinarily go to the left elbow. I omit the upper extremities on the opening and closing spirals and proceed directly from the forehead to the knees on the opening spiral and from the crown to the knees on the closing spiral. I find it preferable to work with both knees at the same time, using my right hand over the left knee and my left hand over the right knee. In this way, one begins to activate the left hand, which is needed in the next segment, after the spiral of chakras is opened. After leaving the crown chakra in the pattern, I recommend the same procedure, using both hands, at the foot chakras.

If you cannot feel the transpersonal point, I suggest that a symbolic transfer of energy be performed above the head to complete the stimulation of the chakras in the spiral pattern.

The next segment, interconnecting the chakras, requires activation of both hands, the left hand as well as the right. One starts at the right foot and right knee. The right hand is held over the right-foot chakra and the left hand is held over the right-knee chakra. One images energy flowing into the right foot and moving in the lower leg to the right knee; then the left hand senses the energy and returns the flow back down to the right foot, and finally one images the energy flowing back and forth between the two chakras in the subject's right leg. When the flow feels free and unencumbered, the next connection can be made.

The chakra connections are made in this sequence:

1. The subject's right foot to right knee, with operator's right hand over subject's right foot, left hand over subject's right knee
2. Right knee to right hip, with operator's right hand over subject's right knee, left hand over right hip
3. Left foot to left knee; right hand over left foot, left hand over left knee
4. Left knee to left hip; right hand over left knee, left hand over left hip
5. Right hip to left hip; right hand over left hip, left hand over right hip
6. Root chakra to lower-abdomen chakra; left hand over lower abdomen, right hand over root
7. Lower abdomen to solar plexus; right hand over lower abdomen, left hand over solar plexus
8. Solar plexus to spleen; left hand over solar plexus, right hand over spleen
9. Solar plexus to heart; right hand over solar plexus, left hand over heart
10. Heart to midchest; left hand over midchest, right hand over heart

11. Right hand to right elbow; right hand over right wrist, left hand over right elbow

12. Right elbow to right shoulder; right hand over right elbow, left hand over right shoulder

13. Left hand to left elbow; right hand over left wrist, left hand over left elbow

14. Left elbow to left shoulder; right hand over left elbow, left hand over left shoulder

15. Right shoulder to left shoulder; right hand over left shoulder, left hand over right shoulder

16. Midchest to throat; left hand over throat, right hand over midchest

17. Throat to forehead; right hand over throat, left hand over forehead

18. Forehead to crown; right hand over forehead, left hand over crown

19. Crown to transpersonal point; right hand over crown, left hand, palm side directed towards the transpersonal point

When making the root-to-crown connection, the energy flow should feel unobstructed between the operator's right and left hands. By the end of the chakra-connecting segment, most subjects' energy fields are balanced and much of the pain that was initially present is relieved or lowered in intensity.

In the next portion of the exercise, the operator concentrates on abnormalities, either those initially reported by the subject or previously unmentioned ones discovered during the scanning. The work is called intuitive because, after relieving the discomforts the subject described at the beginning, the operator allows the intuition to direct the hands in the final balancing of the chakras.

To relieve pain or discomfort in the body, the operator places both hands directly on the area of discomfort and allows a full flow of energy to penetrate deeply into the body. If back pain was the initial complaint, the partner on the table is asked to turn over, so that the hands can be placed directly on the painful or aching area.

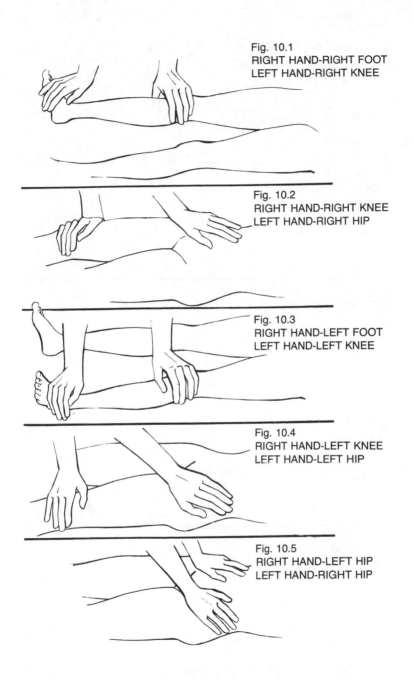

Fig. 10.1
RIGHT HAND-RIGHT FOOT
LEFT HAND-RIGHT KNEE

Fig. 10.2
RIGHT HAND-RIGHT KNEE
LEFT HAND-RIGHT HIP

Fig. 10.3
RIGHT HAND-LEFT FOOT
LEFT HAND-LEFT KNEE

Fig. 10.4
RIGHT HAND-LEFT KNEE
LEFT HAND-LEFT HIP

Fig. 10.5
RIGHT HAND-LEFT HIP
LEFT HAND-RIGHT HIP

The Chakra Connections

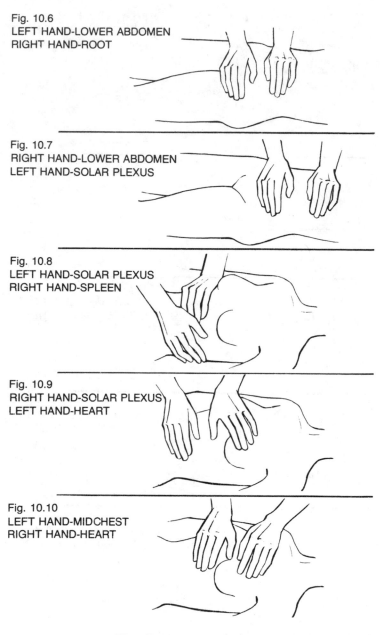

Fig. 10.6
LEFT HAND-LOWER ABDOMEN
RIGHT HAND-ROOT

Fig. 10.7
RIGHT HAND-LOWER ABDOMEN
LEFT HAND-SOLAR PLEXUS

Fig. 10.8
LEFT HAND-SOLAR PLEXUS
RIGHT HAND-SPLEEN

Fig. 10.9
RIGHT HAND-SOLAR PLEXUS
LEFT HAND-HEART

Fig. 10.10
LEFT HAND-MIDCHEST
RIGHT HAND-HEART

The Chakra Connections

Fig. 10.11
RIGHT HAND-RIGHT WRIST
LEFT HAND-RIGHT ELBOW

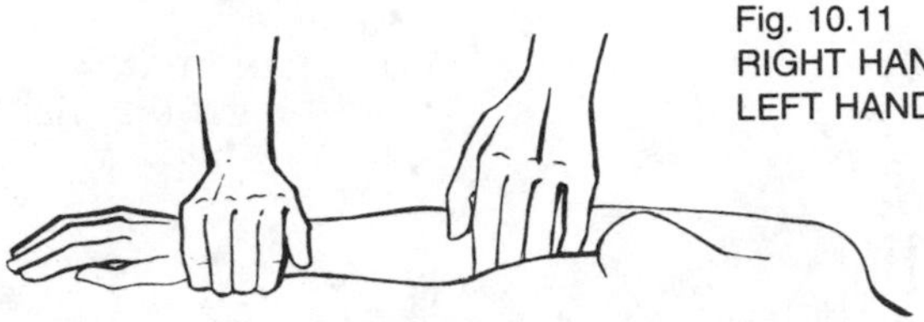

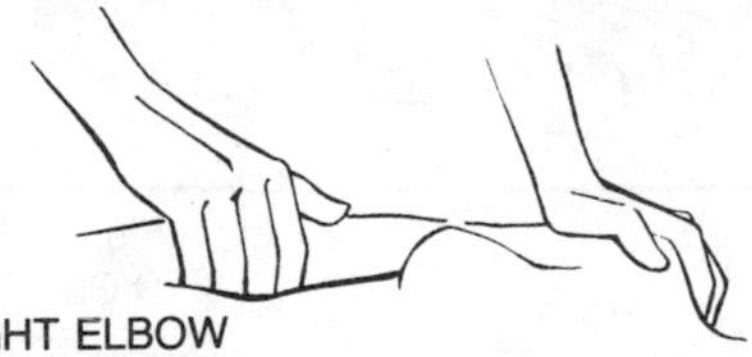

Fig. 10.12
RIGHT HAND-RIGHT ELBOW
LEFT HAND-RIGHT SHOULDER

Fig. 10.13
RIGHT HAND-LEFT WRIST
LEFT HAND-LEFT ELBOW

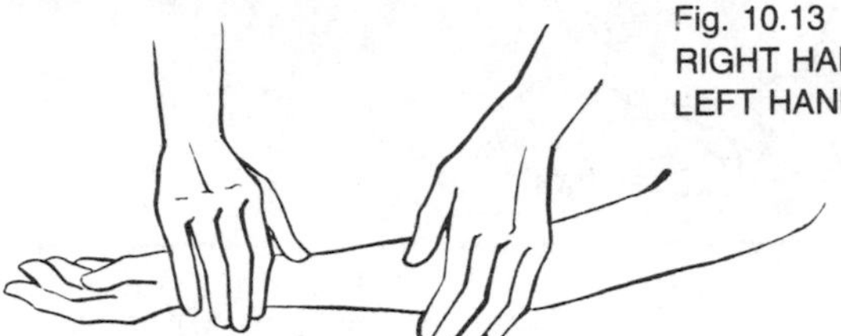

Fig. 10.14
RIGHT HAND-LEFT ELBOW
LEFT HAND-LEFT SHOULDER

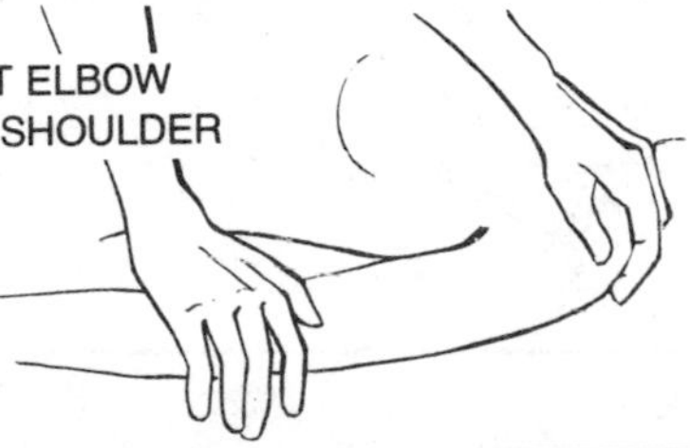

Fig. 10.15
RIGHT HAND-LEFT SHOULDER
LEFT HAND-RIGHT SHOULDER

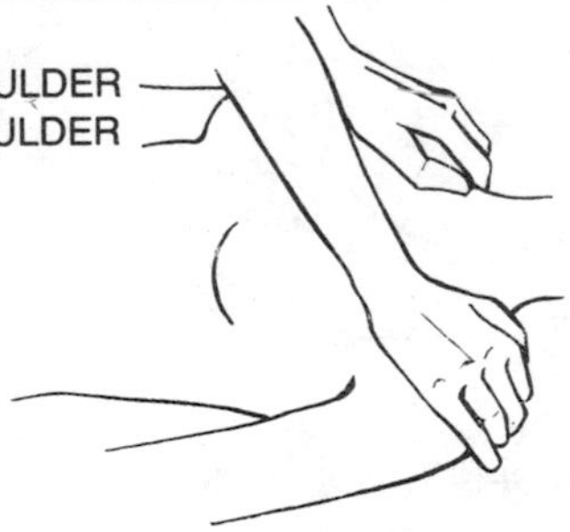

The Chakra Connections

Fig. 10.16
LEFT HAND-THROAT
RIGHT HAND-MIDCHEST

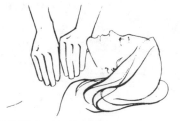

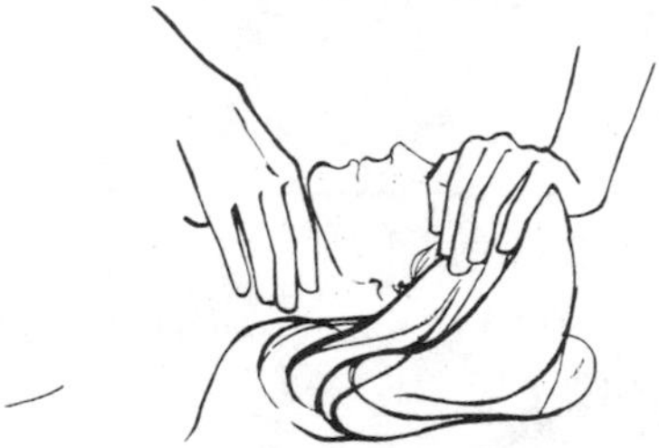

Fig. 10.17
RIGHT HAND-THROAT
LEFT HAND-FOREHEAD

Fig. 10.18
RIGHT HAND-FOREHEAD
LEFT HAND-CROWN

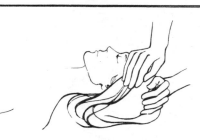

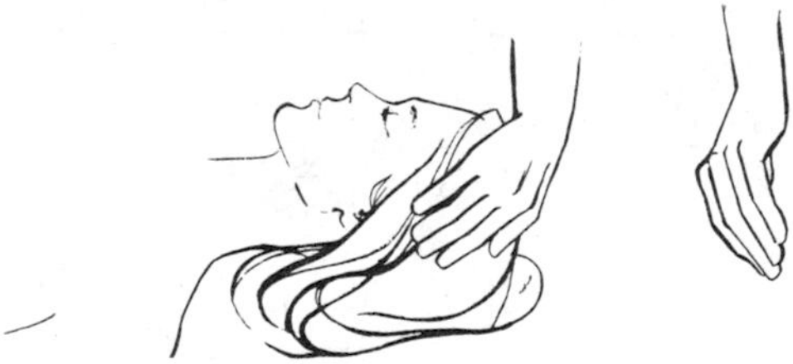

Fig. 10.19
RIGHT HAND-CROWN
LEFT HAND-TRANSPERSONAL POINT

The Chakra Connections

In the relief of aches and pains, the energy flow is turned up to maximum. The operator should feel the hands as intensely ignited—like radiant suns. As soon as a particular pain or ache is totally relieved, the subject signals the operator. The operator does not immediately leave the area, but spends another fifteen to thirty seconds there before moving on. Once all areas of discomfort are relieved, the operator enters the intuitive phase: he or she allows the hands to go where *they* want to go, and not necessarily where he or she thinks they should go.

The operator performs a final hand scan of the subject's body from the crown to the feet, moving slowly and adding energy where it is needed. On completion of this scan, all the chakra fields should feel to be of about the same intensity.

The closing spiral chakra work commences at the transpersonal point of the partner on the table and follows the same sequence as in closing the spiral meditation. In this segment, the operator's hand makes just a brief connection with each of the chakras as the operator feels a deep appreciation for the privilege of being able to share energy with another person.

When the spiral closing reaches the heart chakra, the operator places both hands over the area, lightly touching the clothing and seeking to fuse heart chakra to heart chakra with the subject. The operator holds this connection for several minutes and then consciously and gradually withdraws the energy flow from the hands and from the space between the operator and the subject. This moment is called the "release phase." Unless the operator feels a total release from the subject, a subliminal transfer of energy will go on for an indefinite period of time.

During the entire exercise, the operator must feel that he or she is sharing the best that can be offered, so that at the end of the exercise there is no feeling of noncompletion. If one is offering the best that one can offer at any moment, there can be no such regret as "I could have done it better."

There is no greater gift one can offer than the energy of Unconditional Love.

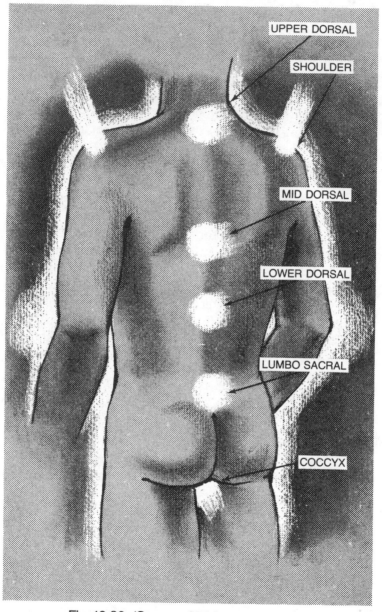

Fig. 10.20. (See pg. 276 for reference.)
The Major Posterior Chakra Fields

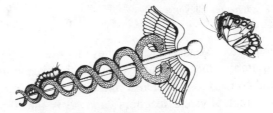

CHAPTER ELEVEN

Transformation

Regardless of the intensity
one cuts wood and carries water both
before and after enlightenments.

The thirteen years I invested in the study and practice of orthodox medicine are now only a fading dream in black and
white, but the knowledge acquired is like the gem called a
peridot: it is clear, brilliant, valuable, durable—frequencies of
yellow, symbolic of the intellect, and of green, symbolic of
healing since ancient times, reflected in the green mantle or
hood conferred at graduation from medical school. Those thirteen years took me to the forefront of scientific and not-so-
scientific inquiry into the harmony and the disharmony of the
physical body and on into the exploration of current theories of
the mind and its aberrations. But neither could teach me what I
yearned to know and to experience—the inclusive awareness
of the body, the mind and the spirit.

A deeper quest led me into metaphysical realms, where the
replacement of clarity by ambiguity horrified my intellect, until
it succumbed to its own understanding of the principle of rela-

277

tive reality. Metaphysics teaches that the entire plane of matter is mutable, that absolutely nothing is fixed unless the human mind conceives it so. Dusk and dawn, the times of change, are great metaphysical teachers, and so is the Tibetan Buddhist teacher, Long Chen Pa, who stated:

Since everything is but an apparition,
Perfect in being what it is,
Having nothing to do with good or bad,
Acceptance or rejection,
One may well burst out in laughter.

One often does. *Humor is the high road into and through transformation.*

A high tolerance for ambiguity reveals options where none seemed to exist before. As ambiguity is accepted, new possibilities of expression and experience emerge as if by magic. One contacts the true multidimensional nature of Beingness.

But my deepest quest led to the spiritual portals brought into view by a radiance of Love emanating through Eunice, transcending the houses of mirrors of both the scientific and the metaphysical. It was, at last, an inkling of that essential Beingness out of which all else is precipitated.

Jumping off the cliff was not difficult. It was a natural progression of unfoldment. Though my mental rigidity offered clarity, it was oppressive, and my Beingness sought release from it. All I had to do was die—die to old traditions, to old models, old methods, old belief systems, old teachers, old friends, old abodes and my own old self. The earlier paradigm functioned well, so long as it wasn't confronted with a deeper intuitive knowing. For systems based on "facts," it is amazing how many facts both the scientific and the metaphysical models choose to ignore. Both systems are valid in a relative sense, but neither is inclusive—at least not inclusive enough for me.

It was both challenging and frustrating, running around in the various created compartments of my mind, keeping track of which thoughts belonged where, which actions were appropriate in any circumstance and which were not, when the irrational could be discussed and when not, conceiving as instructed and conceiving intuitively—and so on and on and on and on and *on*! There comes a time, living simultaneously at many different levels, in many different worlds, when many thoughts and actions seem hypocritical.

But in the central sphere of one's Beingness, it is all resolved — not in any conventional way, not by any "solution" to any "problem," but by the simple fact that the central core of one's Beingness is big enough to contain everything, where apparent conflict does not matter. Here, where there is no time, no cause and effect, conflict can be only apparent; real conflict cannot exist.

In this central sphere, one's Beingness knows myriad dimensions and a plethora of lifetimes—lifetimes where personal and social norms were (or are, or will be) the antitheses of those in what seems to be the present one. When one begins to achieve an overview of these segmented experiences—each always reflected in the pattern of the present life—one must conclude that the fashionable actions and structures of current time are only temporary and are not to be experienced as permanent, and one must at the same time understand that other values from other times may be more dominant in any individual's experience of current life.

If, as I believe, all action, past, present and future, is taking place simultaneously, I must wonder: why should my awareness be centered in this particular dimension and in this particular lifetime? Are they the limit of what my soul can conceive? Am I growing, developing aspects of my Beingness? The task of the Transformational Process is obvious—to achieve again an interdimensional awareness and simultaneously to be in a linear time warp. To me now, the Divine aspects of Love seem to be the solution. To the outer mind, Love may be only tinsel, but to the higher awareness it is a golden thread.

Old traditional patterns are melded into the memory cells.

My life, at this moment, sparkles with creative insight and creative, awakening people. I am surrounded by awarenesses who have varying degrees of access to multidimensional states of Beingness, who are not as trapped in time and space as most, who often see future and past facets as easily as the present, who have identified with the spiritual essence, not its thought form. Fluidity contains the miraculous, and the miraculous is what I experience, not only in the healing of my chronic relapsing pancreatitis, but in experiencing the interdimensional awareness that has instructed and guided my path to this moment. My experience reflects St. Augustine's words: "Miracles do not happen in contradiction to nature, but only in contradiction to that which is known to us of nature."

I am not a completed product but still just a beginner. The four years since I left the practice of medicine seem like a series of dreams in supervivid color, foreshadowing what is to be. There are times when the skeptic in my outer mind becomes enraged at the nebulousness of this beginning, when it prods my Beingness to reconsider the value of this current exploration, when it pleads, sometimes, for a return to security, stability and the conventional. But deeper intuition holds sway, reflecting to my awareness those experiences that can be neither denied nor rationalized as invalid. Tasting a smidgen of the sublime was the first knell of death to the personal self. One finds one's prior existence too constricting, like an outgrown garment. I may not know what is ahead, but I certainly know what is behind. I have no intention of re-forming! The second death knell was signaled by the stirring of the Kundalini energy — the deadly serpent to the ego awareness — as it began to release its preparatory currents.

I sense that the exploration of consciousness, as far as it has been done by the human being, is about as advanced as our exploration of the moon: in both cases, the entire universe is yet to be comprehended. In face of such a vast exploration, I recall the words of a Lutheran minister. They came to him during a group meditation at my home in Los Angeles in 1974. There are just three: "Simplify. Unify. Purify." How powerful these words have become in my life. Of course! The inclusive path is one of simplification, unification and resulting purification. I embrace the simple inside me.

Christopher Fry wrote some wonderfully applicable lines in his *A Sleep of Prisoners*:

It takes so many thousand years to wake,
But will you wake for pity's sake?

Fry is referring, of course, to the simultaneous awakening of both the individual and the collective human consciousness. The "you" he employs is a magical word, because it is infinitely singular and/or infinitely plural, depending on the perspective of the reader. The relationship of the one to the many, the part to the whole, is a matter of current concern to both science and metaphysics, so that one can deeply appreciate not only the influence of the collective state of consciousness upon the individual, but also the effect of an individual's transformation upon the collective state of consciousness.

We are now beginning to experience the result of each of these interactions. As the number of individuals "becoming conscious" increases, a critical intensity of awareness is achieved, and the awareness of the whole is shifting perceptibly: the hundredth-monkey phenomenon is at work. The new collective experience, in turn, seeds greater individual awakening until a sudden jump occurs in the consciousness of both the individual and the group. The miracle is that the jump can occur at all!

For me, the cataclysmic prophecies that are rife in current literature foreshadow a revolution of the most astonishing proportions, but instead of being a revolution in the physical plane it is a revolution in consciousness, a revolution of the mental plane. I sense the approach of a psychological earthquake the magnitude of which has not been experienced in the human awareness for millennia and may not have been experienced in the human awareness ever before.

To one who is fixed in old structures of the psyche, the current changes in thought patterns of large masses of people may appear to be destructive, retrogressive and incoherent. But if one is nearing a state of consciousness that is fluid and future-envisioning, these same tremors of the psyche appear constructive, progressive and coherent. Because I know the potential of my own individual transformation, my excitement now focuses on the imminent collective enlightenment.

Please awake to the potential of your own Beingness!

Sky Hi Ranch
Lucerne Valley, California

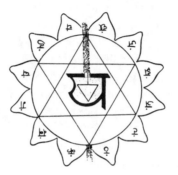

Index